Early acclaim

THE IRRITABLE BRAIN

i

– Kit Campbell shares a brave and inspiring personal journey and exploration of the mind-body connection of living with a chronic illness. The Irritable Brain Syndrome *illustrates beautifully how understanding this connection is the key in the management of our health and well-being. –*
Helena Smetana – General Practitioner, MBBS, FRACGP – Australia

– Words cannot describe how significant Kit Campbell's book could be in potentially improving the human condition on this planet. As a social worker, I daily see the effects of mental disease and the resulting manifestation of negative thinking on the body. The Irritable Brain Syndrome *reminds us of the link between our thoughts and our physical afflictions and builds upon the works of Louise Hay and Eckhart Tolle; empowering people to manifest optimal health in their own lives. I deeply appreciate you for writing this book. –*
Anthony Burke – Social Worker, Counselor – Australia

- Simple, honest, important. Read this with an open mind and heart and relish the opportunity of a life changing prospective. This book goes way beyond its subject. –
Julie O'Sullivan – Travel Writer, Housewife – Australia

– Powerful books come from the strength, vulnerability, and insight of their authors, and Kit Campbell has demonstrated that and so much more in The Irritable Brain Syndrome. *This book is for anyone who has faced a challenge and been crippled by their inability to change their mindset to change the course of their lives. This book is not mind over matter, this is mind on what matters. –*
Troy Hazard – Businessman, Author, Professional Speaker – United States

– I believe that The Irritable Brain Syndrome *is an important contribution to the literature about the power of thoughts. There has been a lot written in this area over the past decade or so. Authors such as Eckhart Tolle and Louise Hay have all asserted the importance of thoughts to our happiness and well-being. However, Campbell's book is unique in that she shows the reader how our thoughts can literally make us sicker and unwell, both psychologically and especially physically. –*
Lisa M. Umina – Award-Winning Author and Motivational Speaker – United States

– All over the world there seems to be a coming together of a greater consciousness/realization that as humans we simply cannot divorce our minds from our bodies. So often when people are ill, a shift in their belief system is necessary for them to overcome whatever affliction they have, guided by clinicians who not only understand medicine but also have insight to how the mind and body interact together. Kit Campbell has been on a personal voyage of discovery and her thoughts and conclusions, set out in The Irritable Brain Syndrome *are enormously insightful and will, I am sure, give hope and motivation to many people struggling with their own health issues, not only gastrointestinal manifestations. –*
Gerry Gajadharsingh DO – Osteopath and Business Owner of The Health Equation – Wimpole Street, London, United Kingdom

THE IRRITABLE BRAIN SYNDROME

KIT CAMPBELL

Originally published in Australia by
Kit Campbell 2012

PO Box 483, Ulverstone, Tasmania 7315
www.kitcampbell.com
email: info@kitcampbell.com

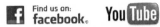

www.youtube.com/user/theirritablebrain

First Australia Printing: December 2012
Second Edition: June 2013

Title 1 of 1 – The Irritable Brain Syndrome
ISBN: 978-0-9874513-0-9
Contributor: Kit Campbell
Contributor Role: Author
Subject: Self Help

Printed by Lightning Source

All I know, is that everything I know,
Is only true in the moment that I know it.

– Kit Campbell

To my brother George:

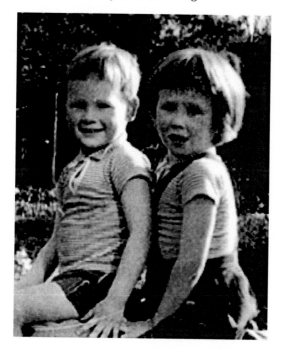

There is no wrong there is no right
But for your life I tried to fight
I tried to take away your fears
I tried to cry your many tears

And now you're gone, I still know you're here
And today one of your shirts I'll wear.
I feel you close and I know you're free
And I'll never lose that part of you in me.

your sister, Catriona

ACKNOWLEDGEMENTS

I am so very grateful to the many teachers and authors I have come across, who have enabled me to share my experience with you. From the beautiful and spiritual teachings of Ram Dass, to the clarity and scientific understandings from Dr Bruce Lipton, and all the others in between. Thank you for sharing your knowledge.

I am also grateful to every person I know, who has given me support and encouragement with each crazy step I've taken through this life, and shared their experience and knowledge with me, to help me along my way.

A special thanks to the academic brain of my wonderful friend and neighbor, who helped me with editing and spelling corrections!

Much gratitude to Helen Bethune Moore, a Senior Editor and Publishing Consultant who has managed to create some sort of structure out of my structureless way of sharing my thoughts, as well as the wonderful assistance of Suzanne Everett of The Bright Print Group, helping me make the final tweaks needed to prepare this special piece of work for print.

Much appreciation also goes to Mark Vernon at Emmark Studios, for all his knowledge and help in getting this book to the hard copy stage.

And I'm forever thankful that my beautiful long-suffering mother is still around to see me complete this project, as she is my number one fan. She may not like every word that I've written, but she will love me anyway. And I love her for that.

Namaste

Contents

THE

IRRITABLE BRAIN

SYNDROME

Introduction

If you wish to upset the law that all crows are black ... it is enough if you prove one single crow to be white.

Psychologist William James (1842–1910)

So, here we are then, you and I.

I am here to share with you my experience of owning Crohn's disease, a forty-year sentence.

Now, I'm going to share another 'sentence' with you that may go against everything you 'know' or have been told by doctors and other 'medical professionals'. *In my understanding, I no longer 'own' Crohn's disease and no longer suffer from it.*

You may believe Crohn's disease is incurable - but I invite you to suspend what you think you know, and read how I cleared Crohn's disease out of my life.

You can keep your understanding of Crohn's disease – that it may be an auto immune disease, or a bacteria that you can catch from a cow – but maybe by the time you've come to the end of this book, just maybe, the key to less suffering could be in your hands.

My hope and wish in sharing my story is that you are able to use my experience for your own benefit. You just never know.

You may have been diagnosed by doctors as having Crohn's disease yourself (CD), or ulcerative colitis (UC) or colitis (C) or ileitis. You may suffer from stomach pain from time to time. Or it may be that you may suffer from fear, anxiety, anger, irritation, frustration, low self-esteem, nervousness; the list of uncomfortable feelings could go on and on! But if you think that you 'suffer' in any way, shape or form, then maybe what I am going to 'share' with you could change the way you use your mind and therefore change the way you 'feel' about things and maybe even change the way your life turns out. Maybe.

Isn't the chance to be free of any form of suffering worth the risk? After all, what am I asking you to do? Just read my story and learn about my journey.

Please note, I am not a medical professional, nor have I had any medical training. Perhaps my training was my suffering and my scars my certificates.

Everything is perception and if your mind currently tells you all I say is rubbish, then that is your perception and you are completely entitled to think or 'know' the way that you do. And if you agree with this, then allow me too to have my perception and my understanding and to share with you and others as to why I believe I no longer suffer from Crohn's disease. And surely less suffering is better.

Now, what I do ask of you is for you to set aside your 'I knows'. Generally, when I share with another, one on one, people will sit in front of me, nodding, saying, 'I know' repeatedly. To me they just know what *they* know and unfortunately, this 'knowing' can prevent new information from being accepted. So just allow my words to be as they are, without trying to make them mean anything with your present understanding. Just catch what you catch and let the rest go.

Along this journey, I will mention the books that I have read, those that have created a profound change for me and the ones I still revisit.

Nothing I 'speak' of will probably be anything you didn't *know* already. I'm not professing to give you the magic solution, or an end to your particular suffering in an instant.

But what I do want to do is to share my journey with you and show you how I turned my health around in a very short space of time. I remember all the ulcer attacks and pain so very well and if someone had told me way back then that I could end my suffering by changing the way that I thought, I would have told them where to 'get off!' in no uncertain terms!

To use a term my brother used, this is not a 'happy-clappy' book. I am not trying to lure you into some religious belief system, or into joining a group. Simply, what I want to show you, is how, one day, after 'owning' and suffering extreme pain, bleeding bowel, yearly hospital stays, many operations, many medications for nearly forty years of my life, the 'disease' I was given to own, Crohn's disease, ended. When I say 'ended', I mean exactly that! I had a few epiphanies along the way – one that involved a washing machine in 1995 (I'll explain later), but the year 2000 brought me the major turning point.

This is when I came across a different way of thinking and a million light bulbs went off in my head. Everything shifted in my mind and everything was different.

At last I realized that the way I used my brain affected my body.

Have an irritable brain, and an irritable bowel won't be too far away!

Chapter 1

In the Beginning

So where do I start?

If you are a sufferer of IBS, CD, UC, ileitis, or colitis, then you are going to want the answer now. And I understand that. I understand the pain, the inability to live a normal life; the pain, as the ulcerated areas of the bowel go into spasm; the pain, as wind travels through your gut, gets stuck and doesn't move for what seems like forever, causing sharp and agonizing pain. The referred pain, in the back and around the kidneys, which makes you wonder if something else is wrong with you. The fatigue, the headaches, the anger and frustration of not feeling 'good'. Being a teenager and the awareness of boys, whilst self-conscious of a bloated belly, not to mention the pain in having sex! The concern about passing wind, which you desperately want to do, but are fearful of passing stools or blood at the same time. The constant worry about where the bathrooms are wherever you go, due to the inability to control bowel motion at times. The thought of having to plan outings or accepting social invitations was always a recurring nightmare.

I've been there. I am no longer there. So here is my story of how I believe it all occurred, and maybe through this, you will find your own answers.

My stomach problems first started at three months of age, going in and out of doctors surgeries with my anxious mother. My first diagnosis of a severe bleeding attack in my bowel was Ulcerative Colitis, which happened at boarding school at 12 years old. At the time, I actually thought I had 'become a woman', as I was told that I would feel a lot of pain and there would be lots of blood. Well, I had both! I started proudly walking around wearing those ridiculous 'hamsters hammocks', as they were called in those days. It wasn't until I started fainting around the place two weeks later, when I got taken to the school sanitorium, where they worked out that I was bleeding from my bowel. I was then immediately rushed to the Radcliffe Infirmary in Oxford and placed under the wonderful watchful eye of Dr. Truelove. What a great name and it suited him too! A year later, 1971, at 13 with yet another bleeding episode, I was re-diagnosed as having Crohn's disease. This was followed with 40 years of suffering chronic conditions up until 2000.

During my adolescent years, I suffered so much embarrassment with this condition and at the top of the list was my frequently bloated stomach.

When the ulcers were festering away in my gut, the peristalsis (the muscular action of the gastrointestinal tract, that moves matter through the intestine by way of contraction and release) would stop and my gut would go into spasm. The trapped matter in the bowel would then give off gas. Gas being trapped in an ulcerated bowel creates unbelievable pain as it distends the bowel.

But anyway, apart from the discomfort, my tummy would extend to the size of a six-months pregnant woman! This made me want me to go and hide somewhere and not to do anything until the swelling had been 'released'. My mother, always the one to come up with a solution for everything, gave me panty girdles to wear! These contraptions were to hold me in and make me look slimmer!

Bloated stomachs are an embarrassment for sure, but nothing compares with the fear of being embarrassed as a result of losing bowel control – even just the thought of the possibility is fear itself.

I remember walking down Oxford Street in my home town of London, on a sunny afternoon, wearing the craziest of outfits, as one did as a teenager in the 1970s, but even crazier as a Crohn's sufferer, for the trousers I was wearing with my fluoro-orange bat wing top, were *white* pedal pushers! You get it? I bet you do. Not the most subtle and safe choice for someone with Crohn's disease. So anyway, there I was, strutting down this high street, when *that* pain hit. I knew that I had around five, ten minutes tops, to find a bathroom. The stress you go through with this is high, and makes the whole situation worse. What made it even worse, was the realization of the ramifications of my white pedal pushers.

But I knew London very well, due to my many temp jobs, and in those days, it was easy to access any building without someone asking you for your blood type and dental records! So my problem was solved quite quickly and even then, I thought that I should write a 'loo' book for London, where to find loos quickly, the best ones and how to go about it. You could never just nervously look around or seem lost, one had to stride in through the door, with an air of knowledge and as a result, no one ever asked questions! But those days of easy access to bathrooms are long gone.

With all the ops I have had, I obviously no longer have a completely functioning bowel. They removed the whole of my left ascending colon, just before the appendix upwards. Apparently, in another little exploration due to yet another 'attack', my ileocecal valve went too. For those who are interested, Wikepedia gives this explanation:

The ileocecal valve, or ileocaecal valve, is of a bilabial papilla structure with physiological sphincter muscle situated at the junction of the small intestine (ileum) and the large intestine, with recent evidence indicating an anatomical sphincter may also be present in humans. Its *critical* function is to limit the reflux of colonic contents into the ileum.

Great! Critical function!

So do I have a normal functioning bowel? The answer is obviously no. Can I cope with what I do go through? Absolutely! It's a breeze, because I no longer have a mental, ongoing battle with a disease. It's gone, because it no longer exists for me.

The White Coat Brigade

Now if you are a medical person, you will probably disagree with my understanding that I no longer have Crohn's disease, as you probably still choose to hold on to the belief that it is incurable. And I totally accept that this is your understanding. For, as I will point out later on, what you know and understand comes from what you have learnt. And if you have learnt that Crohn's disease is, say, 'X' and that is what you believe, then that is what it is – *for you*.

It always made me wonder about medical doctors, when I was being pushed and prodded and tested way back when.

How rare it would be for a doctor to ask you how you feel mentally, or question what has been going on in your life and how are you dealing with that? They seemed to be more interested in what the current symptoms were. They then treat you, or understand your situation, through the words that they have read. This is *past* information. And, as has been proven many, many times, medical information and medication documentation evolves frequently with new evidence. And I used to wonder how many doctors had actually gone through any of these so-called diseases themselves!

I always thought that a fundamental shift of thinking was needed here and happily, it appears that the old way of being a doctor is changing and many doctors are now approaching their patients in a much more holistic way. About time!

To illustrate my present condition after years of Crohn's disease, I would say that it was rather like the result of holding a burning hot coal in my hand. I have now dropped the hot coal, however, the deep scars in the palm of my hand still exist, causing my hand to function in a different way. This is my metaphor for the results of the operations I have endured and the consequent scarring inside of me, which, in the past, has caused me to have further bowel re-sections. Now, it may mean that if I eat a whole jumbo-sized box of popcorn in the movies, that I might find digestion a little hard and uncomfortable! The reason? Popcorn absorbs moisture. The bowel, especially a bowel that is struggling, *has* to be continually lubricated, and this is helped by frequently drinking water. So, if you like popcorn, eat small amounts, slowly and drink lots of water!

A different way of eating definitely helps, especially if you have been subjected to the three-course meal scenario all your life. I will go into what worked for me a little later.

I want to try to explain one's natural state of 'being'.

A fish's natural state of being is swimming around in water. This would make a little fish happy, unless of course he is being chased by a bigger fishy! So now we take the fish out of water and place him on the table. The fish will flip and flop and then start to gasp. He is no longer in a natural state. He is in a state of stress.

So here you are, just being born. You are this tiny, wrinkly, waxy gooey-covered being, expelled into bright lights, ear-splitting sounds, and the pain of oxygen as it rushes into your lungs! Oh, welcome! After being housed in a nice dark and warm environment, food on tap for the past nine months, this experience is a shock to the system and one that will probably be remembered somewhere in the brain's library – this, and maybe the bit beforehand.

There are many thoughts around the awareness of babies in the womb.

What follows is an excerpt from *Sensory Stimulation – Begin the Bonding Process in the Womb* – which is available at www.iamonetruth.com:

As early as the eighth week of pregnancy, the nerve endings that perceive touch have appeared on your baby's skin, and by the tenth week her brain's neurons have begun to form synapses (connections) in response to repeated sensory experiences such as touch and movement. She is already learning as she feels your body bend, walk, stretch, or dance! At about the fifth month her ear is formed, making hearing the first fully functional sense. After this, she can hear most ordinary sounds in the immediate surroundings – voices, music, traffic sounds, etc.

Since the senses gather the information that stimulates the brain to develop, learn, and remember, your unborn baby can be stimulated through auditory, tactile, and movement experiences. Studies have shown that by the twenty-fourth week, baby's heart rate will increase in response to patting or stroking your abdomen!

And consider these two stories from Dr. Thomas Verny, from his book *The Secret Life of the Unborn Child* (2000):

The conductor Boris Brott, when asked when he developed an interest in music, replied, 'before birth'. While learning new music pieces, he was surprised to know certain pieces by heart, particularly the viola parts. His mother, a viola player, was surprised initially, until she realized they were pieces that she had practiced, while pregnant with him.

The emerging fields of pre- and peri-natal psychology are becoming aware of the importance of nine months in the womb, and the birth experience, on a person's physical, emotional and mental health for life. Increasingly, experimental, clinical and anecdotal evidence indicates that consciousness exists before birth, and maybe even before conception.

Not only our talents can come from our womb experience, but also our outlook toward life and possibly certain emotional and physical difficulties. Phyllis Klaus, a psychologist, had a client that had back problems throughout his life. He sought out Phyllis's help as a last resort. In a relaxed state, he was asked to go back to the source of the problem. His body went into a jolt, and he re-experienced an automobile accident while in the womb. He checked with his mother later, and indeed, she was in a car accident while pregnant with him.

Dozens of university and hospital studies show that unborn children can see, hear, fear and perhaps even form a rudimentary level of awareness in the womb. What's more, psychologists now contend that prenatal life and the birth experience are so profound determinant of human personality and aptitude.

So now something becomes a little clearer. If these findings are so, which makes sense, then an understanding of my parents' situation, while my mother was pregnant with me, could be insightful.

Without going into too much biography, I will give you a brief and possible recognizable expectant mother and father.

My father was many things – witty, charming, entertaining, funny and full of stories. He was the epitome of the upper class English gentleman. But underneath it all, because of all the pain he had suffered in his life, both physically and mentally, he could become a very angry man. His escape from himself and his pain was alcohol.

In my understanding, the reasons why the emotion of anger exists come down to one. It is an automatic 'learnt' response to something someone doesn't like – i.e. whenever you bring a 'no' to a situation. Another way of explaining it is non-acceptance to the 'what is'. In the case of my father, it was almost his natural state of being, so one can safely assume that my father's lessons in life must have been fairly harsh and most of those would have come from his father. Behaviors just keep getting passed on. I'm sure being a fighter pilot at the age of 18 years in the Second World War played a large part in that as well.

Please note that although I discuss my parents and their past behavior toward me, I am not apportioning blame. I am simply demonstrating an understanding of how learnt behavior is transferred. Behavior has and always will continue to be passed on, both good and bad, until we comprehend exactly how the 'bad' affects the next generation and decide to fundamentally change this and in turn prevent history from constantly repeating itself.

So, if you respond to a situation with anger, I would say that you already hold anger inside of you. In other words, you have had the experience of anger and have learned how to respond with it. If anyone says anything hurtful or nasty to another, this can only come from their own pain that they carry within themselves. The response is merely the way they have learnt to communicate when feeling that pain. The target audience for this behavior, is always the nearest and dearest. They seem more likely to put up with it.

I remember something Wayne Dyer said in one of his lectures. If you squeeze an orange, can anything other than orange juice come out? Could one possibly extract pear juice, or banana juice? No, because what comes out can only be what is already inside.

I would like to add, that if one were to inject the orange with pear juice, or banana juice, then when squeezed, the contents of the mixture will come out. It will no longer be pure orange juice.

So if a human, when born in its natural state of being – i.e. with joy, wonderment, love etc. and free from any knowledge of pain, anger, deceit, revenge; only an external force/environments if you like, could introduce anything negative, as well as any other negative experiences that may have occurred while the mother was pregnant.

Another person whose work I believe supports this point of view, is Bruce H. Lipton PhD, who began his career as a cell biologist 40 plus years ago. He has written a book called *The Biology of Belief: Unleashing the Power of Consciousness.* This book gives an excellent understanding of cell biology and the mechanisms by which the mind controls bodily functions. Dr. Lipton succinctly explains the cells' functions in the body and what happens when information enters them and how this affects the fetus on a cellular level. More of Dr. Lipton's work is mentioned later.

It's important to understand that everything we have learnt is all locked in our memories, somewhere, so thought and its associated behavior has every opportunity of raising its head from time to time. Even if we 'get it' to a degree, and become enlightened to something, there are still times where the 'animal' part of us, our egoic structure, comes to the fore. In a television interview with the Dalai Lama recently, he actually admitted that he got angry about something! So even the 'divine' among us will still have our past memory of negative and egoic behaviors, our past way of making things mean things, pop up from time to time. This is just recorded information. To use or not to use, now *that* is the question. When you remain still and in the present moment with your mind, you have an opportunity to recognize this past way of thinking and reacting and you then have the choice to let it go with acceptance of whatever the situation is and be who you truly are, to be authentic to yourself.

To me, being authentic to your Self is being who you were when you first got here. My understanding is that when you were born, you had not one bone in your body that had the intention to lie, cheat, steal, to be abusive, threatening, destructive, or any other negative action you can think of. As a fetus or a newborn, you are pure, whole and complete, in whatever form you came in.

When you feel happy, do you feel good or bad? The usual answer is 'good'. The next question I would ask is, when you feel unhappy, do you feel good or bad? The usual answer, although bizarrely not always, is 'bad'. How I see this is that when you are happy, you are in your natural state of 'being'. You are being authentic. When you are unhappy, you feel uncomfortable and therefore out of your natural state of 'being'. This is where you are choosing to be 'inauthentic' to yourself, much like the aforementioned little fishy, happy when in his natural environment of water and not so happy if out of it!

When you keep your mind in the present moment in a 'stressful' situation, you may find the space to ask yourself how you choose to be. Hopefully, you will choose to feel good, then accept the situation for what it is and be able to act with a clear and present mind, free from past reactive energies of anger, irritation, impatience, frustration etc.

You are acceptance, true acceptance. Be this and your future experiences on this planet will be so much more enjoyable!

In reference to my above reflection on the awareness of babies in the womb, I feel that the emotions that the mother 'feels' most definitely have an effect on the child inside.

During her pregnancy with me, my mother went through a lot of stress. Living with my father in a little flat in Edge Street off High Street Kensington, London, could sometimes be a living hell. Walking on eggshells could be one description, but I would say it was more akin to walking in a minefield, as the explosions were often huge. As she felt, surely I would have felt. But how did this manifest for me once out of the womb?

Apparently, I came out crying at 9.05 pm on 12 April 1958 and I didn't stop. Mum said that it was like I was born with a cold, mucous already coming out of my nose. Funny that, because I have had sinus problems all my life and, despite surgery to fix it two years ago, I still have! I've often thought that I carry the world's tears in my head and I don't mean that in any other way, other than having empathy, an understanding that there is a universal suffering, which, when seeing another suffer, we in turn feel their pain.

So, when in the womb, I would have heard the anger, the harsh words of my father and felt the fear, and anxiety of my mother. Once I was out, nothing changed. You come out into this world a complete sponge. You then absorb everything to learn and to gain tools. Everything that is around you, teaches you how to 'walk' through this life. The results of how you use these tools are merely results of learnt behavior. Repetitive learning sets in place your subconscious mindset, otherwise known as the pre-conditioned mind. Check out this excellent book, *The Brain That Changes Itself* by Dr. Norman Doidge. The documentary of this on dvd is really good to watch too.

The child is never bad, naughty, nasty etc. The child, as everyone who walks upon this earth, is pure, whole, and complete. But *behavior*? Now this is another kettle of stinky fish! Behavior is a separate entity that may be unacceptable and ends up having consequences.

I believe it is extremely important to separate the child from his or her behavior. If explained with patience, the child is then able (hopefully) to work out that the parent loves them, but just doesn't like their behavior! This way the child has choice: understanding that if that particular behavior is repeated, then consequences follow.

My parents, especially my father, didn't have a handle on that one. We, my brother and I, were called every name under the sun. I was told that I was "stupid, ugly, I would never have any friends, or if I did, they would only want to be my friend to gain something. I was useless and incompetent and would never succeed at anything." Obviously, there were many times when I would be called endearing names like 'Poppet' and a few others, but funnily enough, I could never remember the good ones so much.

Many times, when 'sharing' with individuals, someone will tell me that they had a 'perfect' upbringing. They were never abused, physically or mentally and that they had a lucky life.

Yet, they are not happy. This can then be expressed in their behavior by way of addictions – ways of escaping the unhappiness i.e. drugs, alcohol, food, sex or work, just to name a few. The body also expresses its discontent, the body being the best barometer for what's going on in your mind, in the form of maybe headaches, stomach-aches, rashes, weight gain, weight loss and so forth. One creates an uneasiness or dis-ease in ones body by the way that one 'thinks', or what you make things mean in this life.

Here's one example.

A woman I knew always had a problem with her weight. She also found it hard to speak up and say what was on her mind. Funnily enough, she had a thyroid 'problem'. As far as she was concerned, she had the perfect family environment. Nothing was wrong with it. She adored both her mother and father; they were perfect in her eyes. She was adamant in her understanding of this picture.

Then, after a little coaxing to find out if there was a significant 'moment' in her life that she remembered, her story came out.

She recalled that when she was very young, her parents gave her a huge accolade by inviting her to the supper table, with the neighbors coming over to dinner! It was the very first time she had been allowed to stay up late and her two younger siblings had to go to bed. She was so excited and felt so special. During the meal, in her excitement, she babbled on about school, and friends, and anything that she could think of. She was so happy. Then a sharp bark from her father, sliced through her effusive behavior. "Will you *please* just shut up, be quiet and let us eat in peace! Or you can go to bed!" Children were obviously meant to be seen and not heard.

This would have been a very significant learning moment for her – one that she carried into her later years and suffered from as a result. If one was to follow the thought process that the minds 'dis-ease' links with the area of 'un-ease', then the thyroid problem could possibly be the manifestation of her fear of speaking her mind when she wanted to. The thyroid gland is located on the front part of the neck below the thyroid cartilage (Adam's apple).

In her book, *You Can Heal Your Life*, Louise Hay introduces a road map to the emotional roots of physical pain and illness, connecting body parts to a variety of major diseases, which is an interesting understanding and I'm sure would have a connection in there regarding the thyroid.

The brain is an amazing processing organ. How it is programmed is how it works. How it works, results in the messages it sends around the body. This is really important to understand. Everything is about what we make it mean and we make things mean things with the tools we were given, i.e. how we were taught to make things mean stuff, like this is good; this is bad. This is black; this is white. This is clever; this is stupid. Then on top of someone else's understanding of how this life is to be perceived, we use his or her tools to look through our eyes and then we start to make things mean stuff for ourselves, with our own perceptions, through somebody else's perceptions... so they are based on no reality whatsoever! Are you now seeing the madness of all this yet?

Once we finally work out that we don't want the results we keep getting in this life, then we have the opportunity to create change. If we don't think there's a chance for change, then there never will be. We must make the choice to change.

These stories that I share with you, also come my own perception. But I share them anyway, in an effort to explain my message to you. You may find me repetitive in places and trying to find different ways of saying the same thing! Hopefully it will be worth it, because the change in my life, due to the change in my thinking, ended so much suffering. I don't mean just from the Crohn's disease symptoms, but also from the space of hell in my mind.

Just to give you a little insight into my 15 year old mind, I wrote this in 1973.

Life to me now is a ball on a string
And mine is hanging loose by a thread
The man with the knife comes closer to bring
The chasm of darkness between the living and dead
The string starts to fray and eventually snaps
I go spinning and swirling down a whirlpool of mirth
Sucking me in to eternity's bonds
As I go drifting away from the living on earth

I used to live in hell and now I live in heaven, yet I'm still in the same 'space' so to speak! So it is true! Heaven and hell are right here on earth! And it's all created through the mind!

Now let's talk about how we make our personal reality through meaning.

Chapter 2

Making Things Mean Things –
The Mean Making Machine

As we walk on through this crazy paving path of life, each experience we have is 'understood' with the previous understanding that we had programmed into us from our parents and peers etc. We then own this knowledge, which in turn becomes our identity and we become very possessive of it. The practice of making someone else 'wrong' and ourselves 'right' is seen in many a conversation. It is simply a battle of identities – another term is 'egos'.

This is such a crazy practice – and one I learnt very well. The one, who 'wins' the argument, feels very self-satisfied, proud of themselves, victorious. But of what? Making the other person feel bad, or angry, wrong? If this person does not understand the practice of acceptance, then the nasty practice of revenge can creep in. And so, it can go on and on.

We can do this without the person even being in front of us! "Well! *so and so*' hasn't rung me in ages! I'm not going to get in touch! It's their turn!" If you want to speak to someone, you simply use whatever communication you wish and contact *them*! Why waste time sitting there and stewing over what you are making something mean, when there could be, and probably is, no reality in your thinking at all! And here is an example of just that.

I remember once going to an advertising industry ball in Brisbane. I had made my outfit out of a white corset and white 'tulle'. After washing my hair, I then set it in perming curlers, to create tight ringlets, which didn't actually work that well, but I did end up with a crazy big hairdo! Anyway, I was working hard to create a 'look'! The make-up on, my friends had arrived give me a ride to the venue – shoes slipped into and the matching bag grabbed, I was ready to go. But I didn't want to wear my glasses, because I felt that it would detract from my intended 'look' so I chose to leave my glasses behind. A little crazy really, as there was going to be a display of award-winning images there and I wouldn't be able to see them! "What about your handbag?" I hear you ask! That consisted of a tiny little purse, hanging from my wrist, big enough for the all-important mobile phone, which in those days, was about double the size of two iPhones, the ever-important business cards for networking and of course the touch-up lipstick.

So, I swanned in to the large gathering, walking '*as a creature like no other*', and had a fabulous night, doing the 'meet and greet' thing, talking about absolutely nothing in particular and laughing a lot. When walking in to a sea of egos, it is easy to float in your own ego boat.

A few years later, I was working on a TV shoot and saw an associate that I hadn't seen for ages. I went over to her and greeted her with enthusiasm. Her body language told me that she wasn't as happy to see me, as I was to see her. Being a fairly direct and up-front person, I asked her outright whether everything was okay. She then enlightened me to the fact that she had been at the previously mentioned industry ball. When she had seen me, she had waved and motioned for me to come over. She said I was looking directly at her, but I then apparently turned my head, turned on my heel and walked in another direction! How rude I must have seemed! How rude she must have felt I was being!

My eyes may have been in her line of vision, but she definitely had not been in mine. I would not have recognized her without my glasses, unless she had been standing within ten feet of me! I apologized profusely and said that I was sorry that she had held on to these thoughts for so long and they were not at all as she understood them.

She said she understood but I haven't seen her since so I will never know.

Isn't it funny how we can make things mean things and get ourselves so upset! But it is also understandable. We will 'read' a situation in the way we were taught to read. How we are feeling at the time will also play a part and if we are used to feeling 'bad', then finding other examples of 'bad' just affirms that how we are used to feeling is normal.

And when we feel bad, we reduce ourselves into it, recoil, or worse, slip down into the deep dark depths of depression, or we escape it with distractions, or we lash out with anger. But I worked out that it's not about how many times we fall down in this life; it's all about how we get back up. The first rung of the ladder is knowing that we have a choice.

As I previously mentioned, my father's escape from suffering was alcohol. So was my brother's, being my father's son. I too escaped my pain, but in different ways.

The messages I got from my father as a child were many, and with each negative experience that I had, my messages to myself became more real.

One of the 'messages' that I took on board was that I was 'not interesting enough'. So to counteract this I would become the extrovert. I would look at all areas where I could express myself outwardly, such as dancing, acting, or singing. Even at a very young age, around seven or eight, I was organizing plays for my parents and anyone else who was around, and charging two shillings a seat. I would write and direct the plays and push my poor little brother around to join in. But I think he too enjoyed the attention. I found it strange that both he and I were born into the same family, yet he dealt with the family structure in a very different way than I did. Also, I believe my father was a lot harder on him than on me – well, this is what I was told at a later time by a couple of relatives.

One day, my father was beside himself with anger. He dragged my brother George and me into the front hall of our house in Kensington. I was made to sit on the bottom step of the stairs and watch while he beat my little brother with a horsewhip. I know that George would have felt more exterior physical pain, but I could not stop crying for him, knowing, once again, that I couldn't protect him and I felt my pain deep inside my gut. It was that old familiar pain of fear – the fear of having no control.

Experiencing the feeling of powerlessness alongside fear, perhaps this is where I learnt to want control so much, because I became so fearful of being at the mercy of someone else. This is where anger is born. Many more experiences were to come my way to strengthen this thought process. Here's a doozie!

My mother and father had gone on a holiday to Ireland for a couple of weeks and my brother and I were staying with our grandparents in Surrey. Whilst over there, my mother suffered a severe kidney infection and was admitted to a hospital. Unfortunately, my grandparents were going away and were not able to look after us beyond the intended two weeks.

While my mother recovered, George and I went into a Children's Holiday Home for around a week and a half. George was four and I was six. We were the new kids on the block, fresh fodder for the previous 'clique' to test and destroy if possible. It was a large house and there were probably eight or nine other kids staying there, two of them being the children of the owners of the house.

For some reason, I became the target for their amusement. I was subjected to, what could now be termed as abuse! I was tied to an electric fence – they laughed a lot at that one! They held me behind a cantankerous donkey and tried to make it kick me! It didn't, but the fear I experienced was huge! They locked me up at one end of a long, low and narrow chicken run and opened up a little gate at the other end. I had to crawl on my hands and knees, through all the chicken poo to the other end, where of course they locked that gate too! They all found this extremely funny. Eventually, they let me out. I was covered in muck and felt completely humiliated. On returning to the house, I was told off for being so dirty and that if I wanted any dinner, I would have to get myself completely cleaned up.

Another trick was, to lure me up to the tree house, with a promise of friendly faces and a game of pretend tea parties. I remember I was wearing a little dress with ankle socks and red shoes, aka Lucy Atwell. Up the ladder to the little house in the trees I went, following an older boy. I got up to the platform, really happy to finally be included in the games. Then, the boy laughed and I looked down to see the others removing the ladder! The boy then easily swung himself down to the ground, taunting me, calling me nasty names etc. I felt so hurt, so embarrassed, so stupid. And as they ran off, laughing as they went, I felt abandoned yet again. The messages just kept on coming, more confirmation. Well, I had to work out a way of getting down. If I were late for dinner, I would get in trouble yet again! The ground below me was covered in nettles. I didn't like them. I had been 'stung' by them before. But I had to get down. It felt so high up and getting out of the branch to swing down like the boy had, seemed an impossible feat. But I gave it a go. I slipped and fell, right into the bed of nettles. The fall didn't really hurt me physically, but the nettle stings were all over my arms and legs, which hurt for ages, but maybe not for as long as how I felt inside.

They did other things too, like tie me up to the bunk beds my brother and I were sleeping in, telling him that if he untied me, they would bash him up. Or, they would hide pieces of my clothing – socks, for instance. If I went down to a meal not properly dressed, I was admonished, and sometimes had to leave the dining room without being fed!

Each of these moments, as all negative experiences that we have do, added to my fear of not having control and affirmed the previously learnt messages of not being good enough, not being liked and never having any friends, unless they wanted something from me. Fear of not having control and being at the mercy of another's cruel amusement. Yuk.

But the worse thing these kids did – the thing that took a very long time to remove from my psyche – was to take me to a traveling fair that was in a neighboring field. Again, they drew me in with promises of friendship and I was desperate to fit in and finally be accepted. They told me that we had been given permission to go and see the fair before supper.

It was very exciting to go on this adventure, and walking off in this group of children, I finally felt like one of the gang. Ah, the sometimes deceitful web we get drawn in to, with that need for inclusion!

We reached the wooden gate and sauntered in. There was noise and color, people moving about, smells of candy floss and popcorn; it was all such fun! But then the next thing I realized was that I was alone! I couldn't see any of the other kids anywhere! Fear hit me hard in my tummy; a familiar pain and my eyes were so full of tears that I couldn't see. I started running around the busy fairground trying to find them. Eventually, after what seemed *ages*, I came to the gate where we had entered the field and I could see a couple of kids and two adults walking up to the gate towards me. They were from the house. And the grown ups looked very, very angry. The kids however, couldn't stop giggling! Kids! It's amazing how cruel they can be! But, as I now understand, they are merely being who they have learnt to be. I held on to this abandonment issue for many years. I recently told my mother of these experiences and her comment to me was, "What on earth did you do to them, to make them act in this way?" Don't you love criticism and blame!

The following is just one instance to show you how my fear of abandonment was carried on through to adulthood, again just showing how these messages received become a way of being. I was traveling from Queensland to South Australia with my fiancé Jason in 2000, and on the way down we visited my cousin Johnny in Bilgola, North of Sydney. Jason had decided to prepare a meal to thank our hosts, so we borrowed Johnny's car and went down to the supermarket to pick up a few things. As Jason felt tired, he elected to remain in the car and I went in to get the supplies. On walking out of the shop, my heart sunk! I had forgotten what my cousin's car looked like, or where I had left it! I looked everywhere but I couldn't see Jason sitting in any of the cars there. And the same fear of abandonment hit me again, causing immediate sharp pains in my gut. I almost felt I needed a bathroom there and then! Please note: This was a physical manifestation of what my brain was doing!

My mind took me into all possibilities. I had known Jason only for around six months and we were already engaged! What if he had stolen Johnny's car and just taken off? These were ridiculous thoughts.

Then finally, after what seemed all of eternity, I saw Jason sit up. He had put the seat down for a quick nap! My relief was not acceptance of this situation and happiness to find him and the car; instead, my reaction was one of anger! And all of this was projected onto Jason directly. Poor guy!

Here I was, subjecting myself to suffering because of what I had experienced in the past and then in turn, turned on the nearest target, Jason, to make him suffer too. My next action was to find a loo.

Here's a story my mum told me about a message she received as a small child, that has stayed with her to this day. Yet another example as to how these ways of being continued through life if not changed. Her nanny had to share her room when they were staying in a small house in Belfast during the Second World War. So that the nanny could come into the bedroom later and turn her bedside light on to read without waking my mother up, she told her to sleep on her right side facing the wall and away from the light. The nanny warned her that if she turned to sleep on her left side, her heart would stop and she would die! My mother has since never been able to go to sleep on her left side and she is now 84! This conversation would have only lasted a few seconds, not even a minute, yet the mind can keep hold of an emotion felt in the moment, i.e. fear, and the meaning making begins and continues until the mind is fundamentally changed.

Like a computer being programmed, each learnt message gets added to our ways of 'being'.

Another message I picked up was that 'I was ugly'. This would then be affirmed by my mother, as she also had low self-esteem. She would always say that her sister was the pretty one. Good story to hold on to Mum! Sad too as this was *so* not the case, not to me.

For myself, my escape was buying clothes. They became the bandages to my wounds, once again ignoring what was causing the wound in the first place. I would charge clothes to my newly acquired credit card (a dangerous thing for a 17 year old!) and feel the rush of owning the 'new' item! Within a very short time, however, the feelings of guilt would creep in and the guilty pleasure would be hidden carefully in my bag, or under my clothes as I entered my mother's front door. I would then rush up to my room and hide it somewhere in the wardrobe. When I would pull the item out later to wear it, my mother, who never missed a trick, would comment "Oh, that's new! When did you get that?" Of course, my guilt would make me feel angry as I found the question to be accusatory, even though that may not have been the intention. So there would usually be a retort of some kind, such as, "I have had this for *ages*!" before quickly changing the topic. This practice and these feelings went on for at least another twenty plus years.

But why the guilt? In my understanding, I learned this from my mother.

My mother was born into a Victorian family, very wealthy and of good standing – the blue blood brigade and all that comes along with it. She experienced World War Two and all the rationing like everyone else and that mentality never left her. Her mother had passed away with breast cancer when she was a young teenager and she then had to look after not only herself, but also her younger sister and brother, while moving wherever their army father was stationed. I would watch her be so cautious with her spending and then show contrition and guilt if she ever bought anything for herself. Monkey see monkey do!

Then there's that time in your life when you start to learn about 'sex'. I remember an embarrassing moment in a classroom once at boarding school while the teacher was out of the room. One of the girls shouted out, "Okay! Everyone who has lost her virginity, stand up!" This was at fourteen years of age for, goodness sake! I remember having to remain seated and then being laughed at. I'm sure half of the girls standing had only experienced an ignorant fumble in their lives, but the peer pressure to be part of the ones that 'know' pulled them to their feet. Why we thought then it was such kudos to lose one's virginity, I will never understand.

When I finally decided, at 16 years of age, to release myself from these 'bonds of virginity', I chose a school friend of my brothers to 'do the deed with'.

I planned the night carefully. My mother was going to be out for the evening, but she knew this chap was coming over to stay at our house in London, for the night. We had many guests stay at our house, especially those who lived in the country and wanted to come into London for the weekend.

Anyway, to cut a not so long story even shorter, the 'moment' happened and it was nothing like what I had read in books, or seen in movies! What a big fat lie! It was awkward, uncomfortable, and painful and I didn't have clue as to what I was supposed to feel! But this being my first time, I thought that it was should be marked as a special moment, so I decided that I should shed a little tear (ever the actress).

The chap saw the tears and asked me what was wrong. It was then I whispered that it was my first experience of having sex and I waited for him to scoop me up in his arms and lovingly tell me how wonderful and beautiful I was. Surely Barbara Cartland, Georgette Heyer and Gilly Cooper hadn't lied to me all those years? But instead, he retorted, 'Bugger off! You're no more a virgin than I'm a monkey!'

With that, he turned over to go to sleep. So, I told him to go back to his room. I was absolutely gutted! What a waste! What a twit I had been! And here I had yet another message to reaffirm my stories of how worthless I was. So, armed with this understanding that sex was a load of bollocks, I went on with my life. But something had changed within me. I had this 'knowledge' now and the competitiveness that had been instilled in me from the word go, drove me on to 'know' more. Couple this with my low self-esteem and the desire to 'feel better', and then add on top of that the realization that I was being 'noticed' by the opposite sex a lot more (or was I just noticing them?) I was definitely going to harness this power of sex and explore it further.

Armed still with the old messages of 'not good enough', along with this newly acquired power, this combination had the potential for negative consequences written all over it.

I changed my 'tomboy' persona to one of a more flirty nature. My head is shaking sadly and slowly from side to side as I write this!

I went to the doctors, got myself on the pill, found myself a 'boyfriend' in the group I had started to hang around with, and my practicing began. I needed to get better at this sex 'stuff', because it was obvious that boys were easy to manipulate in this way, although I didn't really have much of an idea as to what I was doing then.

Then one fateful evening, a negative consequence of my flirtatious behavior came my way. A friend and I managed to get into this nightclub in Tottenham Court Road, under aged at 17. I'm going to cruise over the explicit details of this event and just highlight a major message that I received.

We accepted a lift home from two guys we had been dancing with all night. We had all been drinking alcohol and this of course, separates the mind from the body somewhat. On the trip home, the guy in the back was 'getting off' with my friend and I sat in the front seat with the driver. We arrived outside my friend's house in Holland Park. The driver in the front with me was not to be outdone by his mate in the back and I think he must have watched some film or television show that made him want to live out some fantasy. I was dragged around a corner to a park, Camden Hill Gardens to be exact, and told that if I made a noise, he would make a mess of my face. That line is hard to forget. He offered up a large switchblade as proof. This lesson in sex taught me pain and fear, as I was forced to do things I hadn't even heard of yet. When I finally got back to the house, I just felt numb. I couldn't really understand how people could be so cruel. I must have deserved it. That's what my mother would have said, I thought. I sat in the bath at my friend's house for hours, hoping the hot water would take away the pain from my body and the experience from my mind. I knew I couldn't tell my mother, as she would be absolutely furious with me and never let me out of the house again. Again, the feeling of being powerless was back.

So, I added this negative message to the rest of the others I had gathered. I really was worth nothing. My father said so, my mother let him, and here was life just confirming it all.

So what now? Anger. So much anger, and fear, feeling like I didn't have control of *anything* that happened in my life. So, what was the answer? Attack first. That's the best form of defense. So attack I did. On the outside and definitely on the inside. I started bleeding once again.

Now my mindset here still ran with my programmed understanding, so any realization that my body was reacting to how I am feeling, just passed me by.

And the messages kept on coming. I remember being out with a boyfriend at a party one night. Another girl flirted with him outrageously and it worked. You've got to love alcohol! He started dancing closely with her on the dance floor and the next thing I had to witness, was them kissing each other! Right there, in front of everybody! That added to my feelings of shame. My mind took me right into the place of 'upset'. The good old thoughts came again, "I am not good enough for him. He wants something better." What the thought *should* have been was, "*He* is not good enough for me, *I* should want something better!"

This night had more dire consequences, as the bottle of Spanish brandy, which we had brought to the party, was still half full. I drank the whole lot. I remember being, as they call it, 'blind drunk'. I have a vague recollection of sitting outside on the pavement, being sick and people walking past, asking me if I needed help. It would have been a pathetic sight. I was just conscious enough to be embarrassed about it all and refused their kindness, which, in this case, would have been my salvation.

Then a face that seemed familiar from the party group said that he would give me a lift. So I accepted, as I felt I had no other choice. He propped me up in the back seat of his mini and I remember trying to push my face in the tiny gap that the mini back seat windows have, still vomiting! Lovely!

But we didn't end up at my house, but his. After another episode of being used and abused, I was then shoved into a cab. Miraculously, I got safely home and collapsed in a heap in the hallway of my mother's house, luckily coming to

●

before she found me the following morning. Message to Self, this was never going to happen to me again.

Whatever has happened to this vehicle (my body) is all in the past. I have no connection to that past whatsoever, being here in the present, as the past does not exist any more, so all the more reason to drop any stories I have collected along the way!

The reason I wish to share my many experiences, is to connect with others out there, who have experienced the same or similar and are suffering as a result and to know that there is choice as how to feel about yourself right now, here in the present moment. It's all about choice – to feel good or to feel bad.

But when you think you 'know' everything already, you may not realize that you have this choice. Please free yourself from this misconception. It will be your biggest block. If life here is a constant state of change, then to 'know' will keep you standing still and prevent you from changing your way of thinking and therefore moving forward.

I have finally worked out that all I know, is that everything I know, is only true in the moment that I know it – for me anyway.

Each experience we have can reaffirm the negative identity we have about ourselves, but only if we let it. What we 'know', is also what we tend to seek out in another. And when we see the similarities within the other person or situation, we feel that this is where we should be, what we should be doing, or who we should be doing it with.

But sometimes, you are just in the wrong place at the wrong time.

I would have been around 18 and had been to see a friend, who lived in Kensington Church Street. It was now well past midnight and time for me to get back home to Barons Court. I came down from the flat into the street and looked for the night bus timetables. There didn't seem to be one for ages, so I started walking along the main road, thinking I might catch a cab. It was summer and the evening air was beautiful. I was quite happy walking for the moment and could have easily walked all the way back home. But if a bus or taxi came along, I would take that, as I was wearing these silly platform boots and a knee-length jean skirt that was cut in a 'pencil' style and therefore didn't allow much stride!

I had got as far as Olympia, a good half an hour's trek, walking along the pavement on the left-hand side of the road, when I noticed a man walking on the opposite side, in the same direction. His pace got slower and then he crossed the road to my side, and I could hear his steps closing in behind me.

I almost had a little laugh with myself! "I hope he's not intending to rape me!" God! What a stupid thought to have!

The left turn into North End Road was not too far away and I had started to speed up my walk a little, trying not to show any fear. I was aware that my 'shadow' had shortened the distance between us. There was absolutely no one else around and no cars.

To my left, there were some little shops with awnings. While still walking, I opened my bag and pulled out my keys, jingling them as if I was about to go into my flat. I turned into one of the shop's doorways, hoping the man would then walk on past and leave me alone. He didn't. He came right behind me, his right forearm went across my throat pulling me backwards and into him and his left hand grabbed my crotch. He muttered in a foreign accent, '*Pleeze, pleeze!*' into my right ear.

Now, after the two incidents I had experienced before, I had taken up martial arts, Wing Chun, so that I would never be a victim ever again. Only a year had passed since the last occurrence, but I did have a few classes under my belt and when in the class, I felt confident that I would be able to 'deal' with an attacker, no problem!

That was not the case here. Fear got in the way and the adrenalin coursing through my veins, froze every muscle in my body! I was standing in this doorway, stuck like a rabbit caught in the headlights, for what seemed like forever, with this short stocky foreign man holding me hostage. In reality, it was probably more like fifteen seconds.

Then, from nowhere, my free right arm came up and I brought my elbow down hard and fast into his exposed right side, winding him. As his body doubled up, I then twisted out of his hold to my left and ran. One problem. The pencil skirt! I got away from him as fast as I could, turning left into the North End Road – there was still no one else to be seen – and tottered across the street before I dared to look back.

The greasy little man had sort of recovered and was coming around the corner towards me. His face was contorted and twisted with anger and gave me the impression that he was not happy with me at all!

I was a runner as a kid, but this pencil skirt was holding me back. I stopped, faced him, and pulled my skirt right up on to my hips. He slowed down his pace, probably thinking that I was giving up. I then turned and ran like the wind, finding the first back street that I came to and took off. I knew this area like the back of my hand. This was *my* 'hood! My old paper route! I had to run on my toes, as the stupid boots I was wearing (I even remember the color of them still!) had hollow heels, which made such a racket on the stone pavement, alerting any follower as to where I was! In less than 15 adrenalin-crazed minutes, I was safely on the other side of my mother's front door. Yes, I did have fear, but more than that, I was so angry – so very angry. I also swore off cigarettes for the first time, as my breathing was so labored from the escape!

After this episode my behavior changed dramatically for a while, as my concepts of men were now lower than low, which then became the clouds that distorted my vision. Every man now was not to be trusted, let alone a man with dark hair and foreign features, because my attacker had been dark skinned and a foreigner, so if any man of similar ethnicity dared to look at me, even for a moment, my anger came to the fore without any restraint. But really, it could be any male person. It was very embarrassing for my friends. We would be on a bus, for instance, and some guy might be looking over at us, seemingly to me, undressing us with his eyes. This made my blood boil! My whole body would clamp up, my gut would go tight and it was almost as if I was being blinded by my emotion. I would get up, out of my seat and storm over to the offending voyeur and start swearing at him and telling him to 'go away' using an aggressive and very colorful delivery! I was becoming well practiced in using attack as the best form of my defense. My friends would beg me to calm down and not cause a scene, but this was now my learnt behavior and again, one that stayed with me for many years. So, if someone was rude to anyone with me, let alone to me, my bark was quick and loud and my bite was savage. Now? I feel the old self-protecting ego sometimes appear for just a fleeting moment and then retreat as quickly as it arises. For now I see everyone as 'me', all one and the same.

Looking back, through my choices in life, I was constantly being knocked down. Because of my anger, I was always getting back up, although only to fight, which was not good for my internal system.

My brother was constantly being knocked down too, but he didn't always get back up so easily. As angry a person as he could be, he was definitely his father's son, his action was more of a retreat, with alcohol, which can encourage the dangerous sanctuary of depression.

It's interesting that while writing these recollections of past experience, the memory, held somewhere deep within me, makes me 'feel' a kind of sadness.

A really important point to get here is, not *one* cell of my body that exists today was present going through any of those ordeals years ago. Interestingly though, when I bring the memory from the past into my present mind, it manages to make my body 'feel', as tears can still escape my eyes as I write this paragraph. Placing too much importance on these memories, holding the thoughts in one's mind for more than a few minutes and keeping the meaning, one's body can go through the same stress again with similar physical consequences. Got to watch your mind!

It is so important to let go of the past and not keep dragging it around, which in turn, affects the experience of one's present moment. This is just madness! As I've said before!

Of course, I am only speaking of past negative memories. Once softened and the meaning taken out of them, they can then become just references for us, which may be useful to guide us to better choices.

Thought equals feeling, feeling then affects being.

What also needs to be understood is what the body is made up of. It consists of blood, water, bone, teeth, skin, hair, organs, muscles, tissue and so on. All of these and the rest are made up of cells, which are the smallest units of life that are classified as living things – our building blocks, if you like.

The average life span of a cell depends on the type of cell it is. There are approximately 50 to 75 trillion cells and about 200 different types of cells in the average adult human body. Although some are short-lived, others remain in the body for a lot longer. Let's say you are 20+ years old right now, all the cells you had with you when you were born have now been replaced. An average cell life span varies from a few hours for certain blood cells, 10 days for taste receptor cells, a month for skin cells and 15 years for muscle cells. Although it was thought that the heart and brain could not make new cells, research has now shown this to be no longer true. Got to love changing information!

So physically, everything too changes. A cell is born, it lives, it dies and we leave it behind. Yet, for some reason, we still keep holding on to dysfunctional memory, which seems to drive this ship! The better question here, is *who* is driving this ship?

We have to stop 'knowing'. This is one of our biggest blocks. Just like everything in life there is nothing in science that is static. Scientists are constantly finding new understandings, as a scientist's job is to continually keep testing theories, looking for their predictability!

Yet their 'knowing' also becomes their block to anything they can't prove and sometimes creates a desire to judge another's understanding. Dr. Stephen Hawkins, although a renowned scientist, was quoted by Ian Sample, science correspondent, in *The Guardian,* Sunday 15 May 2011 as saying: "A belief that heaven or an afterlife awaits us is a 'fairy story' for people afraid of death." He himself only understands what he currently understands. This doesn't mean he knows everything. This is just his opinion, not a fact. I would have preferred him to begin that quote with "I believe". Even Einstein was honest enough to state that even though he admitted he was an agnostic, he shunned the criticisms that he was an atheist, as there were still areas of science that are unexplained. As there still are!

Come on! We were once given to understand that the world was flat! The people who believed that, only believed as far as they could see. The same blindfold is worn by those that *know.*

The saying, "Seeing is believing" applies only sometimes and only for yourself and ONLY in the moment that you see it!

We didn't know what an atom was, because the microscope that was being used at the time, could only see as far as the structure of a molecule.

Then scientists worked out a way of creating an even stronger microscope and then all of a sudden, there is the atom! There's something I would like to highlight here. Was the atom there beforehand? Of course it was. It is just that the tool to enable one to see the atom had not been yet created. Much like the new galaxies we are now seeing, due to the telescopes that keep getting stronger. At one point, we thought there was only one galaxy, ours. And now? There's so much more out there to be explored. My point? People should not dismiss the possibility of things, just because it hasn't been 'measured' and deemed a fact by a scientist.

Scientific facts are verified by repeatable experiments, and of course, as hungry as scientists are for new information and a desire to 'test' everything, the atom had to be split in order for them to learn what it was made up of. Enter Ernest Rutherford, a New Zealand-born British chemist and physicist.

Ernest is widely credited with first splitting the atom in 1917 in a nuclear reaction between nitrogen and alpha particles, in which he also discovered (and named) the proton. After that excitement, the rush was then to keep splitting. I believe they have got it down to quarks and neutrinos being the smallest particles 'seen', however, there is no 'thing' inside the atom. It is all just energy.

Another important question, and one they are all dying to quantify, is what is the space between all these energy particles? Now there's a very big question! Why am I telling you all about this? Well, while studying Buddhism, the explanation of quantum physics helped me look at the world in a very different way. It began the fundamental shift in my belief system, which, in turn, helped me to remove the deep-rooted thought processes of dysfunction that I had learnt from a very young age and carried with me for forty years!

And this was the change in my thinking that stopped my so-called Crohn's disease attack dead in its tracks or, if you don't like that terminology, removed all my suffering of the disease or, if you believe Crohn's disease to be incurable, into remission. Whichever way you choose to look at it, I was finally free from the pain and the bleeding and for some reason, I knew 'it' wasn't going to 'get' me ever again.

I think that as a 'searcher', which I feel I have been ever since I could start to think for myself, life can be a bit tiring sometimes, 'going against the norm'.

However, what is the alternative? If you never seek, you will never find. If you just stay the same, keep the same way of thinking, then don't be surprised when nothing changes in your life for the better.

Now, getting back to these molecule things and atoms and so on. Once one understands that everything here of form or what Newtonian physics would call 'matter', *everything*, is made up of molecules, protons, neutrons, and nuclear fission, which are all simply energy, it may start you thinking in a different way. It certainly did me. I am talking about 'form' here and not the space between all form, which is the 'formless'. I need to make something very clear here. As I have just mentioned, there is no 'thing' inside the atom. It is all just energy. The atom is made of energy. The atom is not 'physical'. Atoms make molecules. Molecules are big combinations of atoms, which means they too are made out of energy. Molecules make cells, so therefore cells are made out of energy. A human being is made out of cells, so ... a human being is a collection of energy! Hello! There is no solid mass here of matter! Newtonian physics begone!

So this is what we are made up of. This is the environment in which we 'exist' as humans for the short space of time that we do. This dimension we are all playing around in, is just made out of different densities of molecular structure! Now please don't glaze over here! Just keep 'parking' those 'I knows' for the moment and bear with me and my very basic layperson's explanation of the above which follows!

For instance, you have air, O^2 – two molecules of oxygen. Its density is quite fine, as we can breathe it into our own molecular structures (our lungs), move through it with ease, walking, running and so on.

Then, you have water, H^2O – two molecules of hydrogen and one of oxygen. Now the molecular density of this substance is obviously more dense than air as it is harder to physically move through. It's not 'fine' enough to breathe into our lungs, but we can drink it.

The molecular density of a glass, once heated and cooled, is enough to hold the density of water, as in a glass of water. However, if you were to drop this glass onto a concrete floor, then the molecular density of the concrete would smash the glass. It's not gravity, because if the floor was foam, or lots of feathers, the glass would not break, as the feathers and foam have less density than glass.

To cut through the molecular density of the concrete, one needs an even more dense molecular structure, such as steel or diamonds. And now, new information has arisen contesting that a diamond is the hardest known material in the world! See! What we 'know' keeps on changing! So, we must know that we can only 'know' all that we know in this moment!

Lisa Zyga reported the following on PhysOrg.com on 12 February 2009:

> Currently, diamond is regarded to be the hardest known material in the world. But by considering large compressive pressures under indenters, scientists have calculated that a material called wurtzite boron nitride (w-BN) has a greater indentation strength than diamond. The scientists also calculated that another material, lonsdaleite (also called hexagonal diamond, since it's made of carbon and is similar to diamond), is even stronger than w-BN and 58 percent stronger than diamond, setting a new record.

All of these, and everything else here, is made up of cells, the molecules, the protons, the neutrons, the electrons, and nuclear fission. Everything is vibrating with this energy, but our eyes can only stabilize a certain molecular density. That is, we can 'see' most things in our environment, but we can't see oxygen, for instance. We know it exists because someone has proven it. We can't see gasses, just the distortion of what we can see behind a flowing stream of gas but we know these gasses exist due to the 'proof' of it by scientists.

And so this is it. If your eyes could see all of the different molecular densities, every single 'thing' in your life before you right now, in your room, out in the garden, in this world, in this universe, all of it is just a load of molecules, constantly moving. *Constantly moving and changing.* This is energy and energy equals matter. Einstein's theory of relativity – matter being equivalent to energy, in accordance with its mass, size.

It's amazing to understand, that this mass of cells, all jiggling around individually, are seen as one, for instance re the human, the formation is known as 'the body'. Within this mass is a density of cells which is known as an organ, and given the name 'the brain'. This is much like the mainframe computer and like any computer; information *has* to be fed into it. Once information comes in to the brain, this is then processed and the messages are then sent to the appropriate area of the body.

And then there is the mind. If I were to dissect a human body, would I be able to remove the mind and place it on the table? It's not the brain, that's an organ for the process and storage of information. So the answer is no, you cannot put the mind on the table. The mind is not 'a tangible object. It is not a 'thing'. It is an energy phenomenon. Ask a scientist about thought or about emotion and they will have no *factual* answer for you.

In 1637, the fundamental premise of René Descartes' philosophy was, "I think, therefore I am". That simple statement is meant to be the proof one needs to know that one exists. I think it should be the other way around! "I am, therefore *I* think!"

We 'think' with our minds. Ah! 'To think' is a verb! I think, I thought etc.

Well, the next question that begs understanding here is ... who is the '*I*' that is thinking? *I* am not my mind, *I* 'think' *with* my mind. Yet, my 'mind' is not a physical thing! Wow! The mind must just be an entity, separate to me! That's all! Therefore, being that, *I* should have the power over *it!* Shouldn't I?

And if everything we see, is seen with our own perceptions, then where is the truth? Truth can only be in the mind of the thinker and only in the moment that the thought occurs. Once that moment is over, change has occurred and the truth of the previous moment no longer exists.

The burning question still here is: who is the '*I*'?

Bhagavan Sri Ramana Maharshi outlines it so simply in his teachings, 'Who Am I?' An excerpt from the introduction reads:

As all living beings desire to be happy always, without misery, as in the case of everyone there is observed supreme love for one's self, and as happiness alone is the cause for love, in order to gain that happiness which is one's nature and which is experienced in the state of deep sleep where there is no mind, one should know one's self. For that, the path of knowledge, the inquiry of the form 'Who am I?' is the principal means. (From *The Teachings of Bhagavan Sri Ramana Maharshi* – Translation by Dr. T. M. P. Mahadevan from the original Tamil, University of Madras, 30 June 30, 1982)

If *I* am not my body's functions and *I* am not my organs and *I* am not my mind, which bit of me is really the *I*?

And now we get to the 'space'.

Chapter 3

The Space

What is the space between everything? Between the molecules, the atoms, the subatomic particles of quarks and neutrinos? This space is the field in which all molecular structures 'appear'.

Here I sit, writing to you from my 'space'. There are around 50 trillion to 75 trillion cells that make 'me' up, my hair, my eyes, my skin, my heart, my brain and so on, and there are you and your 50 or so trillion cells. And the space between my cells in this particular mass collection of 'me' here, is the same space that is in between the cells in the mass collection which is you there.

On this planet, within this planet and without this planet – that is, our solar systems and beyond – could the space, the energy that has no name, between our individual molecular masses, including the space within the cells of each animal or human being, be the same energy? Could this be our '*I*'? I believe it could be.

And as much as scientists want to explain this space, many religions and belief systems want to name and claim this space. Some have given names to this space, such as God, Mohammad, Buddha, Christ, Soul, Spirit, Essential Being, Buddha Nature, the Void, the Field etc. Whatever you wish to name it; that is what it is for you. The interesting thing that I understand is that 'it', the 'space', is essentially energy. As it all is. And energy *cannot* be created or destroyed, which funnily enough, is a term used to describe 'God'!

Here are some 'understandings' of this space that I have come across on my journey.

In *The Tibetan Book of Living and Dying* (1998) Dudjom Rinpoche wrote:

No words can describe it

No example can point to it

Samsara does not make it worse

Nirvana does not make it better

It has never been born

It has never ceased

It has never been liberated

It has never been deluded

It has never existed

It has never been nonexistent

It has no limits at all
It does not fall into any kind of category

And Ram Dass highlights this in his book *Paths to God: Living the Bhagavad Gita*, 2004:

> In the New Testament, Luke writes: And being asked by the Pharisees, when the kingdom of God cometh, he answered them and said, The kingdom of God cometh not with observation (not through your senses,), neither shall they say, Lo, here! or, There! For lo, the kingdom of God is *within you*.

This is a common for most religious understandings and each seem to point in the same direction, perhaps just taking slightly different paths. As Eckhart Tolle often mentions, these are all 'pointers'. On this note, I would love to add that Eckhart explains this beautifully, using the example of when talking to a dog! You can tell the dog that the ball is over there whilst you are pointing at the ball. However, the dog will generally look at your hand and not see the ball at all! Too many people get attached to looking at the finger that points and sometimes never manage to get any closer to the Source, the ultimate truth.

If we accept that energy cannot be created or destroyed, then what is thought? Thought *has* to be energy as well.

And, as another saying goes, "As you think, so shall you be." Funnily enough, Bruce Lee, a martial arts expert and actor, was quoted saying the same thing, "As you think, so shall you become." I love it! So many people 'get it' and change their lives as a result. Some understand it, but continue to be the same. And others completely miss it! Another lifetime, perhaps.

Many musicians provide us with so many lyrics that bring a beautiful truth to the table. Listening to David Bowie's 'Hunky Dory' album just the other day, I heard a song I hadn't really 'heard' before, called 'Fill Your Heart' and the lyrics that stood out to me were "Fear is only in your head, so forget your head, just forget your head and you'll be free!" Love it! There's another song, current at the moment, where the lyrics are "Free your mind and the rest will follow!" How true!

So as 'thought' comes in, the brain can then process this information. Within this large electrical component or computer-like system, the brains neurons then fire together, sending electrical messages to the rest of the human structure. The first thing, the thought, determines what these messages do. How that thought is 'wired', is determined by the other first thing – learning how to think.

Now obviously, we are taught *the learning*, in someone else's way, with someone else's perceptions. This is our first hurdle. Outside of our instinctive behaviors, everything else is learnt.

If we are not happy with something in our life, be it our health, wellbeing, work, relationship and so on, surely the first place to look is our mind. How you think with your mind will determine how you feel. How you then feel will determine how you act. And how you then act will determine the results in your life. This is the law of cause and effect, an action and its consequence.

You are not 1 percent responsible for how you were 'programmed', but you are 100 percent responsible for 'being' who you are *choosing* to 'be' right now.

As I have already mentioned, the body is constantly changing, cells just living and dying. The cells in the brain are constantly taking in new information. This is then filtered down into pockets of importance, in a kind of précised version. The less important bits of information are in a less important pocket. (I'm sure that's where all my math studies are!) and the more important bits are closer to the top in a more important pocket. If the brain did not do this, it would become overloaded during one's life and there wouldn't be any room left to absorb any more information. I find this all so fascinating! How cells can live and die, but memory still seems to continue! The reason? Cells have memory. They communicate with each other and pass their information on. Amazing! Listen to Dr. Bruce Lipton on the subject of Epigenetics!

The point I am trying to make here is that *how* you think can be changed. It doesn't matter how old you are, the brain neurons are still firing and creating new neural pathways and will continue to do so until death. This information is supported by the studies in neuroscience and neuroplasticity, and by professors such as Fred Gage in the late 1990s. Gage and his associates showed that human beings are capable of growing new nerve cells throughout life. Before this, the understanding was that the human brain a baby is born with contains all the neurons it will ever have.

Isn't it wonderful how new knowledge is coming forward all the time? The moral of this story is that you can't afford to close your mind to new information and just cling to what you know already. This should now create a great feeling of power within you.

In Sharon Begley's book *Train Your Mind, Change Your Brain,* she writes "Everything we know and remember – indeed, everything we are, our beliefs and values, personality and character – is encoded in the connections that neurons make in our brains" and she tells of a conversation Fred Gage had with the Dalai Lama and other listening Buddhists, where he said, "The environment and our experiences change our brain, so who you are as a person changes by virtue of the environment you live in and the experiences you have."

So now knowing that change is possible and that you do have a choice, what you now need to do, is to look at your 'situation' and work out whether you want to change it.

Sadly, some people seem to be addicted to suffering, constantly finding reasons to complain about something. Eckhart Tolle explains this so well with his explanation of the 'pain body'. (This can be found in his book *A New Earth: Awakening Your Life's Purpose,* 2008. – please read it, a few times!). He describes the Pain Body as a separate entity to one's Self, which needs to feed on suffering! If you have the identity of being someone who 'suffers', then you will either look for suffering, or create it yourself.

Sometimes, if you can't find it, it may be a case of making someone else suffer, so that they, in turn, inflict pain on you. The Pain Body has succeeded in creating the suffering and is now satisfied.

How many of you know someone who continually complains about life, yet does nothing to change it for themselves? Or how often have you seen someone swearing or shaking a fist out of a car window with road rage? (Sadly, that used to be me, *big* time!) Or how many times have you been bumped by a trolley in the supermarket, by someone trying to push in before you at the check out? If you don't react with the anger that they desire from you in order to feed their so-called pain body, they become deflated!

I know this 'Pain Body' so very well. My father passed his on to both my brother and me. Now, understanding how physically destructive reaction is – the anger, irritation, frustration, and so on – I practice acceptance and find it all very amusing. If someone bumps into me with a shopping trolley now, I immediately apologize. The angry face that I first see in the 'Angry Trolley Pusher' quickly softens and then they sometimes apologize too, or walk away in dazed confusion!

I was living in New York for a couple of months, at the end of 2004, while creating photographic images that ended up in my 'Metallic Deconstructions' collection. My first experience of walking on a main street in New York, such as Church Street in Tribeca, was hilarious! Every person walking toward me seemed to look straight through me, striding with such purpose, almost to the level of aggression. Invariably, I was 'bumped into' by many and given such weird looks when my response to the bumping was an immediate, "Ooh! Sorry!" followed by a big smile. I think they must have thought me mad! I, on the other hand, was thinking all of these people were mad! No stillness! No presence! Just people being 'busy'.

Now, even though I 'know' all this and keep connecting with the present moment, I am still tested and sometimes fail! The only difference now is that it doesn't take very long for me to see that my 'ego' has taken over. Once I realize this, I get back to me. Ah, safety!

Driving a car is still definitely my biggest testing ground. I am sure it has a lot to do with how angry my father became when driving! My goodness, he was constantly fuming at the wheel with expletives flying everywhere. You could be quite happily singing away in the back seat, sucking on your opal mints, when a loud, sharp shout sliced through the moment of childhood happiness and fear came straight back in again.

It was like that at mealtimes too. My father was very good at telling stories, always needing to be the entertainer and to be paid attention to. During a story, usually at mealtimes, if he got upset about any behavior that was being practiced at the meal, such as elbows on the table, or slouching, or talking over him, or speaking with one's mouth full, his funny story face was quickly replaced by such a large, black, angry cloud face, which made you feel as if he was going to kill you!

The punishment for speaking out of turn, or with a mouth full, or sucking one's thumb or fingers, was a teaspoon of Coleman's English Mustard shoved angrily into my mouth. The sight or smell of English Mustard today, brings those memories flooding back of punishment, unhappiness and being powerless. Elbows on the table, got a hard knock with a heavy silver spoon right on that 'funny' bone. Slouching merited the embarrassment of a rod or broomstick down the back of your shirt for the rest of the meal! Tilting your chair could result in your chair being kicked out from under you.

Another thing I've realized is that if you eat in fear, it's almost like giving yourself poison. It's so important to keep in mind while eating that you are nurturing yourself with the food and water, and to feel good about that. Feeling relaxed is crucial for a happy gut.

So all the messages that we receive during our life create the way that we think. And as we have already established, how we think is how we will 'be'.

Okay, so we have two choices here in this life: to feel good, or to feel bad. It really is as simple as that.

Please know that you do have a choice. Irrelevant of how bad you think your life is currently, here I am, the 'Talking Pig'. I came across a story about the Talking Pig and I wish I could find it again, to give you the quoted version, but unfortunately it hasn't reappeared just yet, so you will just have to accept my take on it.

A man had a pig that could talk and he wanted to show it off to his friend. I mean, wow! A pig, which could talk? That's amazing! Right? So he called his friend over to meet this phenomenon. The friend did not believe him and came straight over and was introduced to the pig, which said, "Hello," and began to talk. The friend was duly impressed. His next question? "Wow! A talking pig? Do you have another one?" In my understanding here, the friend wanted to know if another one existed for more proof. Really? Did he really need another talking pig to believe that the pig in front of him could talk?

It's much like if I were to go to a gastroenterologist and tell him that I don't have Crohn's disease any more. Here I stand before him as proof, again the one white crow if you like, to prove that Crohn's disease is definitely 'curable'.

He could do tests on me and find me fine, but because of his 'learning', studies and holding the information of those before him, he cannot open his mind to the possibility that what has previously been documented as an 'incurable' disease such as Crohn's can be 'cured'.

So, the specialist's response was always, 'Ah, so you are able to *manage* your disease.' All said with a knowing and superior attitude! They just want you to keep 'owning' your disease: that way, they can keep supplying you with the solutions.

And this is what sufferers would have to go through: sufferers of anything. The medical profession – specialists and doctors – all dealt with our symptoms, rarely going beyond that to find out the cause! Thankfully, more doctors are now beginning to understand how our own thought patterns affect the health of our body.

What is already 'proven' and written down in books is the way it is, right? Wrong! Everything changes, including the information learned at the time of its discovery. Different tests are done further down the track, with different tools and different results are found. Understanding this, nothing should be seen as a rock solid fact and just blanketly applied to an individual in the form of diagnosis and treatment. The 'cause' is the reason the symptoms exist in the first place! Cause and effect, remember?

It is also important for the pharmaceutical industry to keep everything as matter – Newtonian physics – that way they can supply a 'matter' solution (a drug) to a 'matter' problem (your illness). We now know that quantum physics and quantum mechanics are at the core of this universe and all that we know. Another word for this is energy. This is an intangible product and therefore not something the pharmaceutical companies can supply! Imagine them trying to sell you a bottle of energy!

So let's move into the world of pharmaceuticals and the scary relationship between doctors and their drug pushers. Invariably, due to their desire for profit, we become their victims. Rather like bankers and the rest of us in the world!

The 'mind', or how the brain thinks, affects the rest of the body on a cellular level. This has been made so obvious with all the successful results of the placebo.

Chapter 4

I Will Please!

The Latin for 'I will please' is 'placebo'. *That* is interesting.

> The placebo effect is the measurable, observable, or felt
> improvement in health or behavior not attributable to a
> medication or invasive treatment that has been administered.
> – Wikipedia

In plain English, what a patient believes to be a pill
containing medicine to 'cure' an ailment, such as a
pharmacologically active substance, is in fact made up
of a saline solution or a starch pill. This practice of 'fake'
therapies also includes 'fake' surgeries, also known as
dummy, placebo or simulated surgeries! Wow! The trust
we have! You can do your own research on this but here are
some examples. On the BBC site – news.bbc.co.uk – is one
study of these simulated surgeries.

> Researchers at Baylor College of Medicine say their findings
> pose a serious question over the true benefits of procedure
> that is one of the most common treatments for osteoarthritis
> of the knee.

Different groups

In the study, 180 patients with knee pain received one of three types of treatment:

- Sebridement, in which worn, torn, or loose cartilage is cut away and removed with the aid of a pencil-thin viewing tube called an arthroscope.

- Arthroscopic lavage, in which the bad cartilage is flushed out.

- Simulated arthroscopic surgery in which small incisions were made, but no instruments were inserted and no cartilage removed

During two years of follow-up, patients in all three groups reported moderate improvements in pain and ability to function.

However, neither of the intervention groups reported less pain or better function than the placebo group.

And on the *Science Daily* website (www.sciencedaily.com)

Science Daily (July 12, 2002) — HOUSTON (July 10, 2002) Patients with osteoarthritis of the knee who underwent placebo arthroscopic surgery were just as likely to report pain relief as those who received the real procedure, according to

a Department of Veterans Affairs (VA) and Baylor College of
Medicine study published in the July 11 *New England Journal
of Medicine.*

And here on the *Skeptic's Dictionary* (www.sceptic.com)

The idea of the placebo in modern times originated with H.
K. Beecher. He evaluated 15 clinical trials concerned with
different diseases and found that 35% of 1,082 patients
were satisfactorily relieved by a placebo alone (*The Powerful
Placebo*, 1955). Other studies have since calculated that the
placebo effect is even greater than Beecher claimed. Studies
have shown that placebos are effective in 50–60% of subjects
with certain conditions – for example, pain, depression, some
heart ailments, gastric ulcers, and other stomach complaints.

I feel that it is really important to understand this section.
If we have a problem with our health and we go to someone
that we feel is in a position to 'help' us, we want to 'trust'
them, in that whatever they give us medicine-wise, or
organize for us surgery-wise, will make us 'better'. So first,
up, this is about what we believe and the trust we have that
we put in someone who is a qualified 'something'.

As powerful as the placebo can be, it also has failures. And
as powerful as 'medicine' can be at times, this too has many
failures. But unlike the placebo, medication comes with side
effects.

So here we have a placebo pill or 'sham' medication, about which patients have repeatedly expressed relief from their symptoms. So, what's going on here?

Remember the witch doctors? They were very powerful men in the village. You never wanted to get on the wrong side of your witch doctor, or you might get a hex put on you! But, more importantly, the success of the witch doctor is balanced by the belief that the villagers hold for his or her power. If the mind is convinced, for instance, that death will occur on such-and-such a date, the brain could start shutting down the body to the extent that it actually does expire. Or, if someone in the village has a fever and is very sick, in comes the witch doctor, whose energy might create the belief in the patient that he or she will recover, which in turn gives the patient more energy and they hold on, giving the body more of a chance to repair itself. The positive thought energy, I believe, is a fundamental ingredient.

This holds true to many areas today, for people who suffer and look for 'help'. If we are given a pill, or some form of medicine, or a 'sham' surgery and it gives us relief, then surely this is evidence that our minds are more powerful than we know. Maybe it is just the 'giving' or attention from another human being at times.

Many general practitioners will tell you that the lonely or sad clients who turn up to their surgery on a regular basis, just really want to be told, "It's going to be okay."

People visiting a doctor are looking for understanding and compassion more than anything else. But now, a time frame is put on your visit! Go over your allotted ten or fifteen minutes and you will pay more! So don't chat, just get right to the problem and take the medication prescribed for you and then get out of there! I feel that the 'care' part of the health care system needs to be brought back in.

Please note, I would never say to someone who believes that they need medicine, not to take medicine. And I would never say to someone who believes that they need surgery, not to have surgery. What they believe is their truth. But maybe we need to stop for a moment and have a deeper look at the 'business' of medicine.

In my opinion, I feel that a drug is really like a poison, designed to create a chemical change within the body, with the intention of changing the current negative symptoms. This from Wikepedia *"In the context of biology, **poisons** are substances that cause disturbances to organisms usually by chemical reaction or other activity on the molecular scale, when a sufficient quantity is absorbed by an organism"*.

Every drug has a side effect. Sometimes, another medication is given to counteract the side effect of the first prescribed drug! If you go to some websites, such as www.drug.com, you will find a list of side effects as long as your arm with each drug that you search. Underneath the named medication, the first sentence always seems to be:

All medicines may cause side effects, but many people have no, or minor, side effects. Check with your doctor if any of these most *common* side effects persist or become bothersome when using (such and such a drug).

Then, a short paragraph of suggested side effects is given, followed by a longer paragraph of possible serious side effects. Then you can scroll down and find a much longer and in-depth medical explanation of the side effects for the 'professional'.

And yet, desperate people look at some of these doctors, surgeons, or specialists as if they were gods! And they blindly accept the products they sell, often without question and often without looking at the long-term effects of the drugs on their bodies. Please understand that I do not relate this to all of the afore-mentioned professionals, as I have seen many wonderful specialists over the past 40 years or so and have appreciated their professional and emotional assistance.

From the first diagnosis of my symptoms at 12 years of age, I was put on both prednisolone and sulfasalazine. I have since read the side effects of both drugs. It's unbelievable that we take such risks putting these poisons into our bodies! After the many years of taking sulfasalazine, my kidney function, tested in 2010, is now considered reduced. Great! And by giving me prednisolone at the age of 12, not only did it arrest the inflammation in the gut, but also it arrested my development! With a brother achieving 6 feet 4 inches, I could have been a lot taller than my 5 feet 7 inches and had more modeling jobs! My hands and feet are definitely on the large side, which made me feel rather like a puppy yet to grow into its body. Perhaps I should have taken up professional swimming! Prednisolone/Prednisone has since been documented that with prolonged use, especially by children, can result in stunted growth. Again, great.

So just beware the men in white coats and those that 'sell' you their potions. Some are necessary and good for what is needed right then and there and some may not be so necessary and may have a more natural alternative answer. Just for your own sake, do some research and be satisfied that there are no other options. It's sad to think that people opt first for the 'quick fix' of today's candy-doling industry, instead of looking at alternative ways of thinking, or alternative medicine as a last resort, or when mainstream medicine doesn't work.

And that is exactly what I did, before finally turning to seek in another direction. I perhaps should have done it the other way around!

From the age of 17 years old to 33, many life changes occurred – more experiences, more reactions, more suffering, more attacks, operations, and medications, all still fueled by the same old way of thinking. Same thinking, same results.

I got into the music industry in the late 1970s and experienced all that one could in that era. Feeling that due to my 'disease', I wouldn't live long anyway, I lived hard, fast and crazy. Being in the music industry gave me all of that! From coke-infused recording sessions with Davy O'List of The Nice and Bryan Ferry's Roxy Music to working with Clem Curtis of The Foundations and their band, singing back up in London nightclubs. From sitting next to Bob Marley and sharing the green stuff, to jamming all night in basement clubs in Soho, while IRA bombs were being dispersed in the streets above our heads!

As a dancer, I worked on many shows in London and the UK and did a few stints dancing on *Top of the Pops*. Pineapple Studios and the Dance Centre in Covent Garden was a regular hang out during the day and at night, I was always out, dancing in some nightclub somewhere, pretty much every night of the week.

When roller-skating became popular in the 1980s, I worked as a marshal in a roller-skating rink in Hammersmith, The Starlight, which led to a disco roller-skating group, which led to roller-skate promotion gigs all over the UK. We also got picked to be in a Cliff Richard video 'Wired For Sound'! I'm the one in the all-in-one turquoise lycra body suit, with eighties style hair and make-up!

By briefly touching on a few instances in my crazy past, my intention is just to highlight the fact that nothing was ever stable in my life at that time, but it never stopped my drive. Nothing was ever calm or reliable. No thing, no person. The way I lived back then was really a result of the way I felt. Crazy! And in between all of it, my body would still challenge me and when it got bad, I would retreat until I got better, then off I went again. I feel that all of this was me searching for 'me'. Looking for whatever I could find to take me away from the nightmares in my mind – pretty much like anyone who suffers here.

I left my third and last band in 1984, which achieved a number 4 slot in the UK charts, not long after a massive bleeding attack from my lower intestine yet again and more bowel removal. My departure was due to me finding out that my beloved boyfriend had sex with an opportunistic backing singer while away from me on tour – I know, how clichéd! I took myself off to learn the skills of a beautician and in this course, I also learnt make-up application and as a lover of art, took to it like a duck to water. Once I finished the course, I set up my own beauty business in my mother's dining room and wrote songs and poetry when I wasn't working on a client. I specialized in doing nails and facials, but the make-up side of me just kind of shone out somehow. I then decided to go and do a film and television make-up course. I thought that if I could keep adding these varied strings to my bow, then I would always be able to find a job here and there, between my 'Crohn's' attacks. You see, the results of having this reaction to the way that I saw the world, was so debilitating, that to hold down a permanent job was impossible. Whenever the attacks got really bad, I had to hide until they passed. Doubling over with pain – screaming out with it sometimes – or having no control of your bowel movements, just did not fit in to a normal working environment.

I still hadn't 'got' it. I still walked around like an upset waiting to happen! I was still so angry, so reactive, so unaccepting of the world.

On the completion of my make-up course, I went to all the record companies in London and told them I was a make-up artist now and wanted to work on their videos. And I did! It's amazing what happens when you just go for something, knowing you have nothing to lose if you don't achieve it, whatever that something is!

So here I was, back in the music industry, just playing a different part. And it was great! I traveled; I worked with some amazing musicians, such as Paul McCartney, Morrissey from The Smiths, Grace Jones etc., as well as working on film and television, with some awesome actors which included Sir John Guilgud, Sir Denholm Elliott, Dame Joan Plowright and many more. It was busy, it was crazy, it was great fun, but I was still me, still associated with my past mindset.

In 1990, I was invited to apply to go on the Sugar Tax Tour with OMD (Orchestral Manoeuvres in the Dark) as their stylist, so I went up to Liverpool and met with Andy McClusky and he wanted me on board! We toured the UK and Europe, along with Simple Minds, followed by a USA college tour, starting in Toronto, Canada, for pre-production. We did the first show there, then over to Montreal, back over to Boston, and then weaved our way across from east to west, zigzagging to all the main cities along the way. The Red Hot Chili Peppers were doing the same trip just a week ahead of us, and we got to use their band rooms behind them! So messy! But that's rock 'n' roll apparently!

After that tour, I was completely burnt out! That trip could be a book on its own!

My cousin Sue was getting married in New Zealand in December, so this prompted my Australian adventure and next escape. I had always wanted to go to the Antipodes – maybe it could have had something to do with watching *Neighbours* from years ago, or documentaries on the awesome Great Barrier Reef. Or was it because it was conveniently located on the opposite end from the world that I had known? Hmmm. So, in 1990, I left London, with my cousin David, for Australia. I had planned to go for a three-month holiday, but once I arrived, something shifted within me and I knew this was where I was meant to be next. I didn't go back home for three years! My mother was annoyed and my father disowned me, for the second time.

And this is where I met my next teacher, my husband.

We attract like. The rebel in me was attracted to the rebel in him. We joined forces and had fun. But as I've now learnt, one of my many practices was to start something that I almost had no faith in its success or completion. It sounds strange, but the reason was that I could therefore not blame myself when it all went pear-shaped!

So there I was, 34 years old, married, happily enough, to a young chef! He was working in a pizza restaurant and I was working as a make-up artist. We had two very different work schedules and eventually saw little of each other.

Anyway, one afternoon, I was sitting on the floor in our Ashgrove West living room, Brisbane just going through magazines, and Michael was sitting at the dining room table. We were discussing, or so I thought, who would be home the following day to receive a washing machine. Then the sentence that was to be one of major turning points of my life, came across the room, boxed my ears, and made me dizzy with shock! But funnily enough, this moment would be the beginning of the end of my forty years as a Crohn's disease sufferer.

"I don't want a washing-machine, I want a divorce" were the words I heard.

Laughing, I looked up at him, and said, "Don't be silly!" But when I saw tears running down his face, I knew he was being serious.

When my husband voiced his thoughts about wanting to end our relationship, so much fear came rushing through my mind – fear of losing him, fear of being alone, abandoned once again and fear of not being able to control the situation. I felt the immediate familiar pain in my gut, along with the desperate need to go the bathroom.

Two weeks later, my body bled once again, ferociously. And there it was – so blindingly obvious. My body was reacting to my mind.

All this was obvious to me, but not to a gastroenterologist! This is what I don't get! If Crohn's disease is an actual ongoing 'thing', then why do they believe that stress is the trigger for an attack? If it's a disease, why isn't it there all the time? Why can't they understand the possibility that it is the stress that is the 'cause' and the ulcerations are the 'effect' It's ridiculous!

I went to see a senior gastro specialist at the Wesley Hospital in Brisbane, and told him that surely this 'attack' was because I was upset about the impending end of my marriage. This did not go down well at all.

The senior man in the white coat opposite me, sat in his office chair as if it was a throne and spat out, "Don't be so *stupid* girl! You have Crohn's disease! That's all there is to it! Now go away, take this prescription, fill it out, take the medication as prescribed, and keep in touch with your doctor." With a look of annoyance and destain, he turned his face away from mine and went back to his notes.

I was obviously dismissed.

But surely, this is the classic example of 'the process whereby knowledge is created through the transformation of experience'? (Kolb, 1984) Yet nothing here was progressive knowledge at all! My experience was being ignored at the expense of my possible transformation!

This was a significant learning moment for me. Having the experience, to which I reacted with fear, resulted in the bleeding bowel. Looking back, I realized that one experience followed so swiftly after the other. And my conclusion? My mind must have got me into this, so logic begs that my mind has got to get me out again!

I get that there is an understanding of personalities, traits, values and the process of meaning making, as suggested by Morrison (2007), however, I believe that we are born already having some form of experience through being in the womb, as well as absorbing the cellular memory of who knows how far back! Then, to add to the pre-programming, further programming continues once born. As wide-eyed little sponges, we get 'taught' everything – absorbing others' perceptions, until we start having our own. Unfortunately, these are still colored with the inherited prescriptions on our eyes, until we are ready to change that prescription and see the world in a completely different way.

There's another point I wish to raise with this in mind. So many times, I hear that this or that 'disease' is inherited. Have people ever stopped to consider that it is the 'thinking', the 'dis-ease' that is inherited, and not necessarily the disease itself? The body is an amazing barometer for what goes on in between ones ears.

I found this quote on the National Digestive Disorders Information Clearinghouse (NDDIC) website:

While it is recognized that there is probably a genetic disposition in certain individuals for the development of autoimmune diseases, the rate of increase in incidence of autoimmune diseases *cannot be explained by genetics alone* [my emphasis].

There is evidence that one of the primary reasons for the increase in autoimmune diseases in the industrialized nations is the *significant change in environmental factors* [my emphasis] over the last century. Environmental factors include exposure to certain artificial chemicals from industrial processes, medicines, farming and food preparation. It is posited that the absence of exposure to certain parasites, bacteria, and viruses is playing a significant role in the development of autoimmune diseases in the more sanitized Western industrialized nations.

There are other environments outside of the above understanding: the environment that surrounds you at work and at home, emotionally; the environment of sustenance, the type of food and drink that you put into your body, as well as how you are feeling as you eat your meals. But, in my understanding, the most significant environment sits in between your ears! Your mind!

So there I was, walking out of the specialist's office, armed with scripts for more profits for the pharmaceutical companies, a very heavy heart and an extremely leaky head. I think I cried all the way home. It could have been over my marriage being in ruins, the fact that my Crohn's (which I was still 'owning') had come back yet again, or I was just hurt by not being heard. Whichever way it was, I wasn't dead, at least not yet, so why not just try to search for different answers? I did fill out the prescriptions, although I was not sure why. I took the medicines home and placed them in the back of a top kitchen cupboard, way out of sight.

Then my two-year search began.

Chapter 5

The First Steps to Freedom

I had no way of knowing that it would take me two years of searching for an alternative solution to that last attack of Crohn's. For some reason, I just knew that I had to do something different from what I had been doing for the past 37 years. It was obvious that action and consequence played a big part in life, so I needed to be observant of everything that might create a negative effect inside of me. I registered what I ate and drank, the quantities and how often. I recorded whether I had exercised that day or not. I listed the type of clothes that I wore – that is, if I wore a waistband that was too tight around my diaphragm etc. But the one thing that was becoming apparent, the one thing more important than anything else, and that was to be happy! Weirdly simple, but every time I was, there were no problems!

At the beginning of my two-year search, I found myself a doctor who would allow me to walk on this alternative path. She understood my thought processes, and was sensitive to my wish that I didn't want to take the steroids, or any medications for that matter, any more. One stipulation was that I went for regular blood tests to check the levels of both the red blood cells and the activity of the white blood cells, which I did.

Well, I went everywhere and to everyone. The list of sought-out remedies included, food sensitivity tests, allergy tests, acupuncturists, Bowen therapists, magnetic therapy, iridologists, homeopathy practitioners, spiritual healers, kinesiology practitioners, faith healers etc. You name it; I was trying it. I still bled from the bowel every day – every day for two years, but as the time passed the bleeding became less and less as my suffering lessened.

I read that cayenne pepper could be good for the bleeding areas, by the process of cauterization. So, as there was no such thing as cayenne capsules in the early 1990s, I bought some gel capsules filled with some vitamin or other, emptied the contents out and spent hours filling them with cayenne pepper through a paper rolled funnel. Boy! That was fun! My idea was that the gel capsules once swallowed, would dissolve in the desired area! This may or may not have been the case!

I also read that drinking clay was good too! Where I got that information at the time, I can't recall, but some information on the Eytons' Earth website (www.eytonsearth.org) states:

Activities such as drinking clay water, sucking on dry clay balls, and using clay for dental health, is a practice that predates recorded history and spans the entire globe. Evidence strongly suggests that people (and animals) have been safely and effectively using dietary clays for health since before the advent of fire.

So I drank clay. My boyfriend at the time would enjoy telling everyone that his girlfriend had found a new way of getting stoned!

This above remedy will give you an idea of how desperate I was to find solutions, if making my own cayenne pepper capsules hadn't already done that!

During this time of searching for 'the answer', I still worked and played. To handle the pain, I placed hot water bottles on my stomach, which seemed to numb the pain a little. Using painkillers seemed to slow my bowel down, which created constipation, which in turn created more pain, so I couldn't use them.

And then along came another flashing light bulb!

I was on my motorbike under a railway bridge in Brisbane traffic, waiting for the lights to change. A train came along and I got ready to make a wish. My Irish-born mother had always said to make a wish when a train goes overhead, as it will take your wish away and make it come true. Well, I had my wish down pat – health, wealth, and happiness, in that order. The train trundled along overhead and the first word that came out of my mouth for my wish, was *happiness*!

I was annoyed with myself! Why did I waste a perfect opportunity to have a wish come true! But then, this other little voice in my head said, "If you have happiness, then you have all three of your wishes." That was another huge and significant learning moment for me! Some sort of clarity or light seemed to course through me – it was a major 'Aha!' experience! Tears of joy, or relief ran down my face and I rode home with a very soggy helmet!

And as that time passed, things eased and I got 'better'. Or now, as I realize, I became happier. It was almost like I had to go through a period of mourning for my marriage. The loss I was experiencing was more for the life I thought I would have – the forever, the future. This is so amusing to reflect on, as my 'Self' is now so far removed from it all.

So, I kind of 'got' it. If I kept happy in my mind, then I would be happy in my body!

I worked out that alcohol didn't help much, due perhaps to the high sugar content. It was almost like pouring acid onto the bowel lining. Along the same lines as the alcohol, all sweet drinks went out the window as well. So, no more coke, no lemonade, no cordials etc. for me! The high sugar content in coke, ginger beer, or lemonade is amazing! Considering we only need, or will normally use, around ten grams of sugar a day, I believe that one can consume four days worth of sugar in knocking back just one sweet fizzy drink!

I found that drinking water was one of the most sensible solutions for me. If the bowel is well lubricated and less 'sticky', it seems to work more easily. Also, water would hydrate the matter in the bowel and consequently make it easier to pass through and perhaps even the oxygen in the water would help heal me too, as long as it wasn't laden with chemicals. So I started drinking between one to two litres of water a day.

I was also told that smoking was a no, no, as nicotine has negative effects on the bowel lining as well. The lining has all these little finger-like projections called villi and these absorb all the nutrients for the body. The nicotine (the cause/environment) creates mucous (the effect) that can coat the bowel lining in areas, preventing the villus from doing its job. Even though I didn't smoke that much, I thought I'd better give it up completely and give this healing process a proper go.

I tried heaps of different diets throughout the two years. No-wheat diets, no-dairy diets, 'Eat Right for Your Blood Type' diets! The list could go on and on! Sometimes I would wonder what, if anything, I could eat while on these diets!

More information came up about gluten sensitivity, so I continued with a gluten-free diet. Working on film sets was hard, as there was no such thing as a 'gluten-free' meal in those days! I was considered 'awkward' to accommodate with regards to feeding! I wonder if that ever affected my job bookings!

I have also found, that when free from any inflammation in the bowel, I could eat bread and be fine. If I were to choose a particular type of bread, I would go for rye or sourdough, which I now prefer to now bake myself. But I also bake with gluten free flour from time to time.

To aid lubrication in the bowel, a fish oil supplement was also something I used. I don't like to be regimentally taking vitamins and supplements, but if this is something that you like to do, also include vitamin C, which apparently has good healing properties, along with some vitamin D for good measure.

And then there's meat. I'm now a vegetarian for a few reasons. Due to the scarring of past surgical procedures, the most logical reason for not eating meat is that it can be harder to digest than other protein and can line the gut for years! Ask a colonic irrigation therapist! The intestine is important for extracting nutrients out of the food that passes, so to keep the bowel lining free from dead matter can only be a good thing!

Also, when high heat is used on meat to cook it, most of the nutrients/proteins are destroyed! So what's the point?

I would always get the odd meat-eater defiantly defending their position with regards to the fact that humans are designed to eat meat – we have canine teeth after all! I agree. We had canine teeth to rip and chew the raw meat that we ate well over three thousand years ago. We were also probably wearing leaves as clothes, but this too has changed! There were no celebrity chefs around all those years ago; cooking the meat 'man' had caught, delicately seasoning it with herbs and spices! No! It was grab it, kill it and eat it before chummy over the hill could come over and club you for it! Early 'man' didn't have the ability to create fire first up, so meat would have been eaten raw. And there is the use for the canine teeth! I wonder when they did get the first idea of putting flesh into a fire? Hmmm ... food for thought!

But what I now realize, is that no matter what diet I tried, if my thoughts were still of a negative nature, I would continue to suffer anyway.

What follows is an example that describes how the body actually physically changes when stimulated by the brain. It is the lemon story, Wayne Dyer's quote, I found in one of his books. It is a really simple and effective exercise. Try it!

Visualize for a minute a lemon; I've got a lemon right here in my hand. Close your eyes and see this lemon. Hold your hand out and with your eyes closed, see the lemon in your hand. It's got a little nub at the top and a point on the bottom and a little moisture on the outside of the skin and those little indentations like a lemon has. Now hold the lemon and feel it and squeeze it, just slightly. Now what I want you to do is to think of your favorite paring knife, see it, now I want you to take the lemon and place it down on a board and I want you to cut right down the middle of the lemon. Now I want you to put the half with the pointed end into one hand and set the other half of the lemon down somewhere else and just hold that other half of the lemon in your hand. And take your finger, in your mind and rub your finger along the cut side of the lemon at the top, just rub it along the top and feel its moisture, just experience that in your mind and only in your mind, you are all thought. Now take the lemon and bring it up, in your mind, up close to your nose, close to your nose and smell the lemon, smell its tartness and know exactly how it feels and set it back down. Now pick the same lemon up and bring it close to your mouth and open your mouth and I want you to take a bite of the lemon, right here, go on take a bite, chomp! Bite it!

What's happening in your mouth? Do you feel the saliva coming into your mouth? Can you feel it? Just wait another few seconds, can you feel it?

What does saliva do, when acid comes into your mouth? What is the purpose of it?

Feel that saliva fill your mouth!

All through thought. You brought something from another dimension, thought, into your consciousness and made yourself salivate through thought, all through thought, in order to protect your mouth from the invasion of citric acid. That's what happens when you put citric acid into your mouth. That's how powerful thought is and that's what you are.

Were you physically affected by the words and the thoughts of the cut lemon, especially when biting into it was described? Your body physically changed due to an introduced thought of biting into a lemon and there wasn't a lemon anywhere near you! This illustrates how quickly the body responds to your thoughts and therefore, it is so important to be observant of your mind. You need to be able to recognize negative thoughts as they appear, which will enable you to drop them right there and then, before they have an impact on you at a cellular level. Because this is exactly what can happen.

Again, any traditional pharma-medical mind will try to prevent you from believing this, for without you being sick, how are 'they' going to continue making their profits?

And then there's the massive vitamin and health supplement industry too. The hilarious thing is that the pharmaceutical industry wants to make money out of that area as well, by trying to create an accreditation that the product has to pass. It seems they are threatened by the massive growth of the health and vitamin industry over the last 30 years and want to tap into it.

Anyway, getting back to my two-year path. In between all this searching, life continued, work continued and pain continued. A hot water bottle, even in summer, was still my closest friend.

About 24 months along and everything seemed to be 'normal'.

So here I was, feeling like I'd conquered the world! I had managed to escape more medications and had proof that they weren't necessary! For me.

But sometimes enthusiasm can lead one into another egoic mindset. And how easily we forget. I was happier and, as a result, healthier. Work was going well and all thoughts of being 'sick' were far behind me. Old ways of thinking have a nasty habit of creeping in, when complacency comes for a visit.

If you want to be good at something, you have to practice, practice, practice. A professional tennis player will play tennis every day, for at least two to four hours, as will an opera singer sing, or a gymnast train. So, if one doesn't have a continual reminder, with regards to how to think, then past ways of thinking come and take over again.

Ever the entrepreneur, I was, as usual, always thinking up different business ideas! One was to start a virtual art gallery, with unique art pieces that I could travel the world finding. I came up with a name, a business plan, and found a three-level warehouse in Kangaroo Point, on the river in the city center of Brisbane and set about bringing this idea to fruition.

The cost of the warehouse was $220,000 (a mere drop in the ocean in comparison to today's prices) and it came with a tenant that had a long lease. I was going to keep him on the lease, but reduce his expenses by using one of the levels for my studio. It was all so exciting, all so encompassing and then all so overwhelming, and I was once again reminded as to how damaging my mind could be on my body.

Bringing this product together and worrying about finding the finance etc., the pressure I managed to create for myself was enormous. My mind wouldn't stop thinking and planning and trying to work out how to achieve it all. I was doing it all on my own, as usual, and worry and fear crept on in, with the old messages and stories of "I'm useless, I'm not good enough, I'm a failure, I will never succeed in anything."

And here we are again. As sure as eggs is eggs, my bowel started bleeding. I was so frustrated! I didn't have another two years to fix this! I wanted it fixed now!

I had a chat with my gastro specialist, Dr Graham Radford-Smith, at the Royal Brisbane Hospital, who told me that I would probably be looking at more surgery and definitely another bout of steroid treatment and that I should take this seriously, as bowel perforations can be deadly.

So, I regretfully booked in a pre-surgery appointment for two weeks time. I had to abandon the warehouse and art studio project, as it wasn't going to come together financially with only me behind it and there was no one else interested in backing me.

At the beginning of the two weeks leading up to the hospital appointment, I had a job doing make-up and hair on a commercial. During the day, when the models took their breaks, I noticed that one of them didn't join all the rest of the others in their usual chat about what they had been working on lately. She was sitting crossed-legged on the floor in a corner, reading a book. I found myself intrigued at her non-interest in the model social circle and walked over to discover more.

I asked her what she was reading and I was then introduced to a Buddhist type belief system, called Falun Dafa.

Now, just as a reminder, I need to repeat that everything we come across is just a pointer, guiding us to new understandings in this world. If we just get stuck watching the finger that points, then that is exactly what will happen to us. We will be stuck! Remember the dog and the ball example?

The model gave me her book to read and although I hadn't read a book in almost ten years (didn't have time, too busy, too many things to do, people to see, whatever!) I gave it a go. I started to read a page or two before going to sleep and a page or two before getting out of bed in the morning. At first, reading this book was hard as my ego was still being very strong, but then, for some reason, it became so easy that it was almost like a light continually going off in my head! Within seven days of reading this book, all the bleeding in my bowel had stopped. And that's no word of a lie. A fundamental shift in my way of thinking had started to happen.

The strange thing is, if I read the book, *Zhuan Falun*, again, it no longer points to where I currently am. In fact, it seems not to sit well with me at all now. I don't mean Buddhism itself; I mean the actual book *Zhuan Falun* is no longer 'right' for me. It was merely the pointer to take me from where I was to where I was meant to go next.

It's quite bizarre! It's like the simple concepts of Buddhism, developed over two and a half thousand years ago, spoke to my Western mind and cracked open all the ignorance that had built up over the years I had been here on this planet.

It's obvious that Buddhism was aimed for the people who were around at that time and the message of having nothing and owning nothing is probably not going to be accepted by the Western people of today's world. But that's not the message I got.

The message I got is that it's the attachment that needs to be removed. This comes with acceptance. We can 'have' things around us in our lives, as long as we have the understanding that there is no permanence. Every thing at one point or another will dissolve, including us!

One minute I have a precious ornament intact, the next it might be broken on the floor. If I have attachment to the ornament, sentimental or otherwise, then I will suffer. If I have acceptance, when the ornament breaks, then my suffering is minimal and this gives me the clarity to act, whether it be cleaning up the mess and throwing it away, picking up the pieces carefully and maybe putting them back together again, or whatever.

I wasn't taught any of this as a child. I watched as my father ranted and raved when things went wrong in his life.

He taught me that angry non-acceptance was a suitable reaction to just about everything. My mother had her opinions of what was right and what was wrong and, as a result, could be very opinionated and critical. This again is non-acceptance. I noticed that being critical was another bad trait that I needed to drop. My criticism of another could never determine how that person actually was, it just determined that I was someone who criticized!

Well, I was dropping these learned traits left, right, and center! And as a result, I was becoming lighter and lighter! All I could do all the time was laugh and cry and sometimes both at once!

I attended my pre-op hospital appointment the following week, and I remember the walk on the way there so well. I had tears welling up in my eyes constantly, followed by the odd giggle! My goodness! Anyone looking at me would have thought me insane! But then who are the sane ones?

And there I was, before the specialist, who knew me quite well, luckily.

I told him that I no longer had Crohn's disease and that I was never going to suffer from it again. He was very accepting of my earnest manner and said that he still wanted to do the examination.

The examination done, Dr. Radford-Smith was actually satisfied. He told me that it seemed I was presently doing well. However, if any bleeding was to occur again, that I was to immediately contact the hospital and come straight back in.

I felt like shaking him, not in an aggressive way you understand! I wanted to make him understand what I knew, that I no longer had Crohn's disease and that I would never be 'coming back in' again, but I didn't really know how to express what or how I was thinking! It was all so new, hard, easy, complicated, and obvious all at the same time!

I sailed out of his office on a cloud!

So, here I was, this new little 'happy clappy' as my brother would have called me! I was so overjoyed at this new understanding, that I completely immersed myself in Falun Dafa, studying the lectures old and new, repeatedly. I joined parades all over Australia, as well as in Hong Kong and New York, to bring awareness of the 150,000 Falun Dafa practitioners, who have been wrongfully jailed, tortured, put in labor camps in China. Amazing, isn't it! If something or someone becomes popular through speaking their truth, the current power either harnesses it or crushes it. Much like how it would have been for Jesus, who was crucified, or the Dalai Lama, who had to flee his own country.

Needless to say, many of my friends thought I had gone barking mad! They were happy for me that I was well again, but couldn't stomach my constant smiley face!

One major corner stone, was going to the back of that kitchen cabinet and pulling out all the drugs and medications and throwing them into a bin! I had elation mixed in with a tiny serve of 'Oh my god! Am I really doing this?!' as their existence in the back of the cupboard had been a type of psychological cushion - the 'just in case' factor.

As my effervescent reaction lessened somewhat, I settled back in to life, but for five years remained studying Falun Dafa and being sexually continent, a term Ram Dass once used for being celibate, and both drug and alcohol free.

But then I started to notice that even though other practitioners were studying the same thing, they would sometimes twist the understandings of Zhuan Falun to suit themselves. That was just my observation and opinion. I would also see egos still working away, as well as normal human manipulation. I was beginning to become aware of the boundaries of this particular understanding, and it was then I realized that *all* belief systems, including religions, had boundaries!

In 2004, I wanted more of challenge in my life. I decided to buy a ticket from Sydney to New York and out of LA back to Sydney, take my camera with me and promised myself to shoot at least one image a day. So off I went, to spend a very cold December in New York for a couple of months. While I was there, I went to a couple of peaceful presentations performed by Falun Dafa practitioners. It felt good, but for some reason, more questions were entering my mind about in which direction I was to walk next. But, funnily enough, you never really need to ask a question for very long as things just turn out the way things are meant to be.

I got some great shots while in New York and met some awesome people, but the weather was doing me in, it was so cold, so I jumped on the net and bought a seat on the next plane out to LA, where I was going to live in North Hollywood with an actress friend of a friend.

During my two months in LA, I did some work with a headshot photographer, doing make-up for her, as well as doing some headshots of my own. I found that my body was beginning to send me messages again! This time, it was in the form of a hernia in my left groin! Luverly!

Now this had started as a very small 'bump' before I had left for my trip and I had approached another Falun Dafa practitioner and asked her opinion as to whether or not I should have it 'fixed'. The answer came back as no, for it was just karma! And karma should be removed by being a good practitioner, through meditation and the like! The Falun Dafa understanding was that if one was to have an anesthetic, then all the good 'energy' that had been cultivated within, during one's practice, disappears!

So, this is an understanding that became a boundary for me and one I felt I had to cross. *Zhuan Falun* was written by a Chinese man, Li Hongzui, in 1982. I'm a white Western woman right here, right now. I felt it was time to go with what felt 'right' for me.

With the bulging hernia, I was now finding it hard to walk without pain. It was time to put a plan of change into action!

I contacted a hospital in Melbourne, booked the op with a specialist over the phone, changed my return flight date out of LA back to Australia and off I went on my next adventure!

My beautiful mother-out-law (she used to be my in-law!) took me under her wing and we used one of her holiday vouchers to stay at a hotel overlooking the bay in Melbourne. The operation came and went and I was bulge free!

So now I had the hard job of acknowledging that I felt I could no longer 'call' myself a Falun Dafa practitioner. It was incredibly sad and I shed many tears over my decision. I just felt that anyone who said they followed anything, a religion or a belief system and their scriptures, yet just did what they wanted to do, was a hypocrite. It's similar to when a person calls themselves a Christian, yet is a racist; or when someone who calls themselves a Roman Catholic, sins, because they can go to confession later and be 'forgiven'. That confuses me! Surely we have choice over what we think and therefore what we do? People who swear, or cheat, or steal, or commit adultery, or rape, or take a life, or take advantage of their position in life over others, and then go into a church once a week, or once a fortnight, or once a year at Christmas and call themselves a religious follower of 'anything' is something I cannot understand.

My fellow practitioners tried to get me to change my mind, telling me that it would be okay, and that I would be able to build up my 'energy' again through practice. But I had made up my mind. Another path was becoming clearer and I needed to walk in my own shoes for a while.

Once I had made the break; that was it. I hardly heard from anyone! One minute I had this large family supporting me, and the next I was an orphan, an outcast! I think they might have been worried that I might infect them with my desertion!

I absolutely understand why people like religion or belief systems or groups of any kind. It creates the feeling of inclusion, involvement, and the confirmation that you are on the right path – that what you are doing and thinking is okay and accepted by others. I think many lonely people go to churches every week, just to be with others and to be accepted by them, which is good. It's all about what you get out of it. That's also why some of these new churches are so successful with the youth of today, bringing them in through music, and increasing a sense of belonging which, in this fractured world, happens less frequently, as parents seem to have less and less time to offer their young.

But whatever works. The same messages seem to run in each religion and belief system; it's just that the separation of the belief systems create problems. Separation is not good. Not any type, as we are all one and the same.

So now I was feeling a bit lost. No real direction as such, but I knew another adventure was just around the corner! As I've now learnt, practicing standing nowhere is a very safe place to be.

I was still determined to keep the three elements of Buddhism within me always – truth, compassion, and tolerance. Very simple, very beautiful.

More tests for me were just around the corner and were going to test my new way of thinking to the max.

So, 2005 was slipping away. I was no longer an 'anything'; just me, back in this crazy world alone again – a little sad about it, but feelings of euphoria also buoyed me up, like there was 'more' to come, but I just didn't know what or how. Then the next trigger came.

Whilst looking in the mirror one morning, I noticed, what I thought was chocolate on my night T-shirt, just a few drops on the right. I didn't think much about it, until I noticed more of these spots on the left-hand side of the T-shirt the following morning - yes I wore it again! I investigated further and noticed that the T-shirt was inside out. The 'spots' were coming from my right nipple. It was dark-colored blood.

The mind immediately popped up. My right breast is not well! What's going on? But this kind of 'inner peace' was still with me and this quiet logic just gave me a clear mind and no tight stomach, as I looked for a doctor's number to make an appointment. I'm sharing this with you, to show you how, by practicing 'acceptance' of any situation, you are then free to act, with clarity, without distress.

Before I knew it, I was sitting in front of a breast cancer specialist in Wickham Terrace, Brisbane.

A whole flurry of x-rays and blood tests happened the following day, and the day after I was being prepped for a lumpectomy, to check out what was what. At the same time, the surgeon was kindly going to take a test of a small mole on my stomach that a skin doctor didn't like the week before. I thought I might as well have that checked out at the same time.

Every time my mind slipped into those negative speculations of 'what if', I reminded *it* that I was now in the world of the 'what is' and refused to pay attention to anything outside of the 'now'. I was fine right now! All I had was a leaky nipple and a dodgy looking mole!

A couple of days later, I was out on the balcony of my apartment, being the assistant to a friend, who was building a wooden screen around it for me. The phone rang. It was my specialist telling me that yes, I did have breast cancer, which had to be removed straightaway after the weekend. I was booked in for Monday. Ah. Okay. Right! My mind was beginning to whir away, creating a bit of a head spin. "Oh and by the way," the surgeon added, "I've got some bad news, I'm afraid." Well! This should be good, I thought! "That mole we had tested, was malignant, Stage 2 melanoma. It needs to be completely removed, immediately. We will do that at the same time." Fabulous! This day was just getting better and better!

After I had put the phone down, I really tried to make sense of all the words that had gone into my ear and all the words my mind was throwing at me. Amidst the confusion in my head, I managed to realize that right now, like I was before I got the phone call, I was fine! I felt fine. So what had changed? Only the information. How was I then going to deal with that information? Well, that bit was up to me.

I thought that maybe I should be hysterical! Or devastated! I actually couldn't believe I was asking myself, "How should I be feeling right now?" Before, I would possibly have been totally re-active and emotional, for that was how I had learnt to 'deal' with moments in life that were unpleasant or unacceptable!

I walked back to the balcony and told my friend the news. He was more affected than I was! It all seemed a bit of a dream really. I felt that I was supposed to be really upset, and tell everyone, so that they could get upset with me. That now seems a bit bizarre!

But the 'what is' was that I had a balcony job to help with, so I just carried on working away with Matt.

When I told two good friends about it the next day, they rushed over, with ice cream and movies and sat with me in complete silence, escaping into the celluloid dream. It was almost like they didn't want to talk about 'it'. I really did, in a factual way though, but went with the flow of the moment, as maybe to talk about 'it', would have upset them.

So the operations came and went. All the 'bad' breast tissue was removed, along with a fairly large amount from the 'bad' mole! In fact, the mole removal wound took longer to heal than the breast wound did! No chemo or radiation, for the breast cancer, I didn't want that. In my understanding, chemotherapy and radiation kill cells, both the bad ones and the good ones. If my surgeon was happy that he had removed enough of the unhealthy tissue and its surrounds, I was happy. I didn't need to sabotage my body any more than that.

My friend Matt brought me over a disc with around four public speakers on it. They were Byron Katie, Wayne Dyer, Marianne Williams, and Eckhart Tolle.

I started listening to the first two speakers and I enjoyed what I heard. I found that listening to Marianne Williams challenged my understanding with, what I perceived to be, a high level of Christian religious talk! I moved on from listening to her quite quickly.

I didn't listen to the last speaker, Eckhart Tolle, I thought his name to be a bit weird at that time but concentrated on the first two. This is now funny to remember, as Eckhart Tolle is a wonderful gateway to understanding and enlightenment. But I feel that everything happens the way it does, when it does and maybe I needed to be introduced to the first two, in order to be ready for Eckhart! I was going from an Easterner speaking his understanding of Buddhist scriptures, to Westerners speaking their understandings. But it was an easy transition.

As I was listening to Byron Katie and Wayne Dyer speak at their recorded seminars – really beautiful simple stuff – I saw a similarity to what I had already studied with Falun Dafa. Yet this was different. It was giving me tools and not boundaries. It was expanding my way of thinking, and using my mind in a much more healthy way. Life was just getting better again! I was happy to find other people, who had similar understandings as I did, explained in a more Western way. These again were all just pointers. I don't think there are any 'words' that can really be followed, much like any 'one' or any belief system or religion. Everything has boundaries, this is what creates the identity of something; therefore, if you want to continually surpass your knowledge and understanding, you cannot get yourself stuck on anything, anyone, or any individual belief system or religion. That will just keep you within that system.

Anyway, I got better from the breast and skin cancer surgery and time marched on.

It seemed that throughout my life, I was being made aware that my body was also my teacher. This was something I was told when I was 14, by a well-known homeopath in London. I remember asking her how come I was suffering from this Crohn's disease so young, as everyone else in the clinic in Fulham's Charing Cross Hospital was so old?! She told me that my journey was the important factor; what I was going to learn by having the disease. I had no idea what she was talking about then, but looking back now, she spoke so much truth.

It was also amusing, as even though the way that I was looking at the world was continually changing – and for the better, the 'tests' I was having didn't reduce; they actually increased! It was almost as if an external source, was saying, "Right, so now you think you've 'got it', we will just keep helping you test that theory!"

Most of the 'tests' are the small sneaky ones, when you are not paying attention to your ego, as it judges the person in front of you for a moment.

How can you judge? Who are *you* to judge? Pay attention to your ego and it gets back in its box pretty quickly.

The next test, a very big one, brought me closer to an even bigger test. And the journey continues.

Chapter 6

The Journey Continues

At the end of 2007 my beautiful brother George, who lived in London, was diagnosed with stage 4 cancer. He was deemed to have six months to a year to live. This was devastating news. He was someone I had tried to protect for so long, but had to give up trying and finally left him to the fate of his own hands and those of others around him.

I had one more breast cancer check up appointment to keep and then I would fly to the UK in eight weeks time, to be with him and my mother. I also had my tax to sort out and as I wasn't sure how long I was going to be in London, so I thought I'd get that done and out of the way. My out-laws were away and I took this opportunity to go to Noosa and housesit for them and look after their newly acquired dog, finish off my tax, then come back, have the check up and fly to London to be with my brother.

While I was in Noosa, I accessed Matt's disc again and for some reason, clicked on a video of Eckhart Tolle, one when he was speaking in India.

You know that feeling you get when something gives you amazing clarity? It's like someone blowing peppermint through your brain. It's all cool, clear, and breezy! I felt another fundamental shift in my mind and the following two weeks were spent doing my tax, walking the dog, and listening to Eckhart every moment along the way. Every jumbled thought that I had, every bubbling emotion of anxiety and fear in my gut, just seemed to fall off the shelf. Almost like a bedroom that is absolutely covered in mess on the floor, on the bed, and in the cupboards, and then Mary Poppins comes and clicks it all away! It was awesome!

I still had great sadness in me, but it was no longer clouding my mind, filling my gut with lead, blinding my eyes with the hot anger of blame, and making my body ache with pain from the impending loss of my brother George.

I went back to Brisbane after the two weeks housesit and with my flights all booked, started getting sorted out to leave.

George had been given chemo treatment. But not satisfied with just one hit of the poison, 'they' decided he needed another treatment.

I managed to Skype with him once. My mother was concerned about how I would react, as he had lost a lot of weight during his ordeal. When I saw his face in front of me, I barely recognized him. And then he spoke. And then I saw him! "It's so good to see you!" I effused, bubbling over with happiness at being able to talk to him in person. George, like my father, hated speaking on the phone and any phone conversation you did manage to get with him, was always very short.

"You're beautiful!" I said. George laughed and replied, "Are you sure you're looking at the right person?"

"Absolutely! All I can see is you! It's like your house might be a little worn here and there, the paint peeling a bit, but your light is still on and shining brightly and is beautiful to see!" My family has had to put up with my 'happy-clappy' attitude over the years, so they were used to my 'funnyisms'.

The conversation was short, but I felt like I had been given such a special moment that was huge!

Two weeks later, just before I was due to fly over, I got a phone call from my mother to tell me that he had died.

After I put the phone down, I just sat on the sofa and a low load moan came out of my body from really deep down. I don't know what it was, but I could really feel part of me howling. There was no thought as such involved, just an expression of loss, I guess. Daze followed, and clarity was gone for a little while. There are those stages of grief – funny how everything seems to get categorized. But the one thing that got me through it all was listening to Eckhart's philosophical teachings. Accept the 'what is', the present moment, and then act.

I was asked to read at George's funeral and had a set amount of time in which to speak, so while waiting for my flight date and during my trip, I wrote my piece for him. I shed many tears along the way, but as I mourned his passing, this beautiful peace stayed with me. I had already gained this clarity; life just brings along things that cloud it from time to time.

Now the first thing that usually happens when a test like this, breast cancer etc., comes along, is that my stomach gets all tied up in knots and the next thing I know, I'm having bowel problems. But through this different way of thinking, I am able to see that when my mind creates the negative past thought process; I can then release the thought before it causes me a negative physical result. It's not something that once realized you can forget about! It's a matter of constant observation, making sure the mind stays a friend and doesn't revert back to being a foe.

Going back to London, to the funeral, was going to be a hard test. But the two months that involved dealing with my mother and her grief, along with clearing up George's flat, and his life, that ended up being a huge test.

Each time I came over to visit my family, especially my mother, certain relationship 'issues' were sometimes overcome and surpassed. Some, and some not. But with this trip, I felt, the fractured relationship between my mother and me was about to change, for the better. I was different and I had different tools. But it was definitely no walk in the park!

Grief makes people angry in the middle of all their sorrow. Being in such close proximity of each other for two months, there were moments where nearby targets got hit. My spiritual way of speaking annoyed my mother from time to time and she lashed out left, right, and center. My past self-protection mode was desperately trying to kick in and get me to lash back at her and then run – far, far away!

I had to be very mindful of my own perceptions and my past mind creeping in, whispering, "If only you had... Why couldn't you have...? Why didn't you...?" etc. Hello *Blame*.

I had spent many of my early years trying to protect my brother from my father's anger. Then, when he was 14 years old, I tried to protect him from himself. This is when George began drinking heavily, sometimes a whole bottle of gin or vodka in a day. I also had to protect him from my mother. My mother was playing the part of the enabler well. She rationalized that his drinking was because his father was no longer in the home and the head of the household, and my brother was feeling 'lost' as a result. Therefore, as I was the oldest, he must feel displaced. Huh?! I left home soon after that; as I made what my mother had said to me mean that his drinking was due to his 'displacement', which was due to my existence. And therefore due to me. My mother, would not accept that he had a problem and that he was an alcoholic. She just said he had a 'drinking problem'. She would excuse her purchases of Sainsbury's low alcohol beer for him, because there was hardly any alcohol in it. Never mind the fact he could drink 20 or so cans of the stuff in a session, or drink the whisky from the bottles under her bed, then fill them back up with water! Ah! The sweet blanket of self-deception.

But we got through it. Two months later, we were still both sad, but something had been healed between us. I would even say that my mother was beginning to shift in her way of thinking. And for me, I found another level of acceptance of her way of being. After all, if we don't accept the 'what is', then we'll just go insane! It's the only logical way of getting through this life isn't it?

So, life goes on. These large holes of loss in life that we experience don't go away, but as long as we can stand beside them and remember, rather than fall into them and despair, we will be all right.

Every time a well of emotion, usually a feeling of loss, comes up, you just observe the swell in your body. Just observe it. You can feel it, but don't 'be' it, if you know what I mean. Thich Nhat Hanh spoke beautifully about these emotions – how you can 'hold' the emotion like a baby and give it love. Hold it apart from you, and don't make it a part of you.

My mother possibly fell into these holes more heavily from time to time. It was hard for her, considering that she and my brother George lived together, on and off, until he was in his forties. My brother was so similar to my father that the time they spent together gave her familiar comfort and company at times. Once again, she had someone to need her, which she seemed to need herself. She possibly felt it was her raison d'être. Another way of explaining this need to be needed, is codependency. Another tool I used to own.

As people get on in life and become more static in their home, old memories are often used to entertain themselves and shared with others.

Well, my mother loved going back into the past. However, she couldn't really grasp the fact that most of the things we remember are how we *perceived* the happenings in our lives. We then create beliefs about these happenings, with our perceptions and our stories then unfold, with very little reality in them whatsoever.

And all my memories are just that too – memories. Not only memories, but *my own* perceptions of what happened. Holding on to some of your old negative thoughts can bring past negative emotions back into the present, continuing anger and frustration, sadness and bitterness. And yet, the situation does not currently exist. It no longer exists, yet how many of us drag past perceptions into the present and live in hell as a result? How many countries are at war, wasting countless lives, and spending massive amounts of money that they should be using to feed, clothe, nurture, and educate their people, all because of things of the past? Insanity!

If we want to choose to feel good, if we want to choose a happy life, there are just two words needed here.

Stop and *it*!

Stop and It

What is it about this feeling of anger and revenge towards another? How come it actually feels, in a *very* weird way, kind of good?

Is it the adrenalin rush we get that runs all over our body, or is it due to the blood rushing to our extremities, our arms, legs and head, a tingling sensation is felt? Or is it that opportunity to be right and make another wrong, bringing a sense of winning, feeding the ego? Whatever the reason is, the speed with which anger can take over is scary. Heard of the saying 'blind fury'? This is when the mind goes into 'protection' mode and uses instinct, instead of going in to the rational part of the brain and using intelligence. So one could say that when one is angry, one is less intelligent! So finding the space just before the rolling stone of emotion gathers momentum is a good place to step into before it runs us over completely.

How long is it going to take before we realize that when we hurt one another, we only end up hurting ourselves? By continually bringing our past perceptions into the present, there's a very good chance things are going to go wrong.

These memories, our past perceptions, don't go away; they don't 'go' anywhere. They just sit in the cup, the mind. Our job is to filter out the good from the bad. Ignore the bad memories in the cup and enjoy the good ones from time to time.

And this is what we all need to be very aware of. The bad thoughts can creep in at any time, hence the importance of being the Observer of the Mind! This gives you the opportunity to choose the good and not the bad.

One analogy I came up with to illustrate this involves a tennis court, a tennis ball serving machine and you on the opposite side of the net. You have a bat in one hand and catcher's mitt in the other. The machine is filled with green tennis balls, as well as red ones. With the mitt, the idea is to catch the green ones. With the bat, this is to hit the hell out of the red ones, right out of the court! Yes, the green ones represent the good thoughts and the red balls your 'bad' thoughts. Where should you place your attention? At the machine! This way, you will 'see' the color of the ball being fired out at you and this will tell the mind to choose the hand holding the bat or mitt to come into action. What could happen if someone comes up to you on the court and wants to have a conversation whilst this is all going on? Immediately, your attention (your conscious mind) is diverted, so your subconscious mind takes over the batting and the catching. And here is where the problems of not batting and catching the right balls can occur! If the subconscious mind is wired with negative thoughts, you may find yourself catching the red balls! And if the wiring you went through, told you that you didn't deserve the good stuff, you may find yourself batting the green balls out of the court! I don't know whether this 'worked' for you, but my intention is to show that you are the batter and the catcher and the tennis ball serving machine is your mind.

Chapter 7

The Next Test

My next test to put more of my new skills into practice, came the year following my brother's death.

In June 2009 there was a family wedding happening back in the UK and my mother wanted to attend, so I went to London to take her and spend some time with her, as well as to catch up with family and friends. We went to the wedding but Mum was not particularly well at the time. She had the beginnings of a bladder infection. On top of that, it was quite cold and windy on the day, but she insisted that she was fine and didn't want to wear a shawl I had brought for her, as she felt it was more important to socialize in what she was wearing and freeze! Ever the one to keep up appearances!

By the end of the third week of my visit, the infection took its toll. At 4am an ambulance had arrived at the house to take mum to the hospital, as her temperature was seriously high and she was being sick. I remember pacing around in emergency, waiting for ages before someone would come and attend to her. Her body was burning up, but her teeth were chattering, as if she was freezing. She was no longer communicating with me and her whole body was shaking so violently at times that I thought she was going to have a heart attack and die. As much as I may know now, my past way of coping with things can sometimes come to the fore and my use of anger popped up. I remember doing that looking-up-into-space thing and saying, "Not now! Don't take her now! We still have so much more work together yet to do!"

I then became more vocal about my concerns and demanded to see a doctor. I offered up the possibility that should my mother die in their emergency waiting room, out in the reception area for goodness sake, without care, that they would be looking at a negligence lawsuit! I really had no idea whether that was the case, but something must have registered as a doctor came out and mum was then taken to an emergency ward and treatment started. After about two or three hours, probably around 7am, color was coming back to her face and she seemed to be more coherent. The bizarre thing was, she had no recollection whatsoever of going in to this state. I, however, was feeling terrible at seeing her suffer yet she wasn't really even suffering herself. Weird! It must be that somewhere in our brains, we shut off, like a self-protective mechanism.

After a couple of days in hospital, she looked much better. I was due to fly home to Australia in two days, for two weeks of back-to-back shooting. I didn't really want to leave her, which was a revelation for me! But Mum insisted that she was in good hands and all would be fine. She was on intravenous antibiotics and therefore had to remain in hospital. After that, she would return home.

So, I reluctantly left her and caught my return flight back to Australia.

A week and a half later, I found out from my neighbor – yes, my neighbor and not a family member – that Mum was very sick, and back in hospital again with yet another infection. In her email, the neighbor told me that if I wanted to see my mother before she died, I needed to be on a plane very soon. Major shock! What is this that I'm going to experience now? My brain was rushing yet again into the future!

What was the problem? Unbelievable as it may seem, the 'safe' hospital space had given her a gastrointestinal bug – Clostridium difficile, while treating her for the bladder infection she had actually been admitted for. This was a very dangerous strain of a bacteria, highly resistant to antibiotics. Many elderly people, as well as infants, have died as a result of contracting this bug.

My mother didn't want me to know and had avoided telling me. I rang the hospital and got the facts, rang my mother and got her perceptions and told her I was on my way. I then worked on getting my thinking straight to keep myself present and sane, packed a bag and got myself on a plane, again.

So here I was, in another stressful situation. While in this state of stress, even though I was practicing hard, listening to my lectures constantly, knowing that I can only do what I can do, knowing that I can only feel what I 'choose' to feel, unfortunately the cortisol (stress hormone) that my brain was producing, was beginning to affect my gut. As much as we think we 'know', knowing is not the key. *Being* is the key. Wow, I've still so much yet to learn. Awesome.

Cortisol, the name derived from *cortex,* is a hormone in the body that is secreted by the adrenal glands. It has been called 'the stress hormone' because it's also secreted in higher levels during the body's fight or flight response to stress and is responsible for several stress-related changes in the body.

Small increases of cortisol have some positive effects, such as a quick burst of energy for survival reasons, heightened memory functions, a burst of increased immunity, and an ability to lower sensitivity to pain.

While cortisol is an important and helpful part of the body's response to stress, it is also important that the body then relaxes, so that its function can return to normal following a stressful event. Unfortunately, if the stressful moment is prolonged, without the balance of relaxation, the body has no chance of returning to 'normal', resulting in a state of chronic stress within the body.

In 2012, Elizabeth Scott, on www.about.com, discussed stress and stress management and defines the difference between a short burst of acute stress and the prolonged state of chronic stress:

Chronic stress is a state of ongoing physiological arousal. This occurs when the body experiences so many stressors that the autonomic nervous system rarely has a chance to activate the relaxation response. (We were built to handle acute stress, not chronic stress.) This type of chronic stress response occurs all too frequently from our modern lifestyle, when everything from high-pressured jobs, to loneliness, to busy traffic, can keep the body in a state of perceived threat and chronic stress. In this case, our fight-or-flight response, which was designed to help us fight a few life-threatening situations spaced out over a long period (like being attacked by a bear every so often), can wear down our bodies and cause us to become ill, either physically or emotionally. In fact, it's estimated that up to 90% of doctor's visits are for conditions in which stress at least plays a role.

Some would say that it's very important to learn stress management techniques and make healthy lifestyle changes to safeguard you against the negative impact of chronic stress. I would agree and then add that this is where 'acceptance' needs to be practiced on a continuous level, so that when a possible 'stressful' situation arises, there is no reaction. Just action.

Scott gives further examples of how being constantly stressed, or keeping chronic levels of stress, negatively affects the body.

- Higher and more prolonged levels of cortisol in the bloodstream (like those associated with chronic stress) have been shown to have negative effects, such as:
- Impaired cognitive performance
- Suppressed thyroid function
- Blood sugar imbalances such as hyperglycemia
- Decreased bone density
- Decrease in muscle tissue
- Higher blood pressure
- Lowered immunity and *inflammatory responses in the body*, slowed wound healing, and other health consequences.

I am so grateful that there is more acceptance of the many ways the body is affected by how the mind is dealing with a situation in 'life'.

Now we can see that prolonged stress leads to high levels of cortisol in the body for long periods of time, which leads to inflammatory responses in the gut.

Well, sorry, Doc, but don't 'give' me the title of Crohn's disease! That's just a name! If you take away the name of Crohn's, the title of the symptoms, what would you say is going on? Answer? An inflammation of the bowel lining. What's inflammation? An inflammatory response in the body. So the next question should be what is the *cause* of the inflammatory response? Stress. And should we now have a look at why the patient is in a constant state of stress and help them work out how they might change this for themselves? Yes!

Understanding how the brain can affect the body on a cellular level, surely, it is of the utmost importance that we pay more attention to how we think.

All you 'I knows' out there; you need to stop doing that, for the sake of your own health. Understand that everything is change, and please keep parking your past and your past ways of knowing, and allow new information to come in. Now this might change how you saw things in the past and you might feel that this challenges whom you thought you were/are. But surely, if life is change, then shouldn't we be and think with a constant element of change? Our body certainly is! As has been previously established, not one cell within you right now was there at your birth! Everything has lived and died within you on a constant daily basis, so surely your 'I knows' should be dropped and your present understandings allowed to create change in the way that you think.

Some people would find this all too much. And that's okay. You can come and go here as much as you want; you have all eternity to keep working it out!

I guess to challenge someone's identity of who they think 'they are', because of who they 'have been' can be hard for someone who is attached to the past. To me, this is suffering. And there are those who still wish to suffer. Everything is choice. Ah well.

Again, as I mentioned before, all that I am 'knowing' now, can get kicked in the butt by my past knowing if it pops up and takes over while I'm not looking!

A reminder of where you need to be is always good. And where is that place?

Right here and *right now*. In this space, everything is tangible. So, each time the 'fear' thoughts pop in – fear being a negative emotion about something in the future that hasn't even happened yet – it has to be released by bringing oneself into the present moment. Some do this with meditation, removing thought. I find that a good tool is to 'get present' physically. Touch something, your chair, your clothes, etc. Feel the texture, the temperature of what you are touching. Observe all that is around you, what you can see, what you can hear. Observe your breathing, breath going in, breath going out. This is mindfulness. This will keep you present.

Chapter 8

Mindfulness and Minding

There are monks who do a walking meditation. It's called the practice of mindfulness. This is being focused on what is happening right here in the now, with no thoughts present. As you pick your right foot up, you sense the muscles in your leg working and as you place your right foot slowly on the ground, you bring your attention to the connection of your heel to the solid surface and then to the rest of the foot. Your awareness senses your body moving forward and then you bring your attention to the left leg as the muscles move and the left foot is lifted from the ground. And so on. This is a very peaceful practice and one that can calm the mind quickly, but only by releasing your thoughts and changing your focus of attention. You may find your mind interrupting you, like an annoying child whining, "Think me! Think me! Think me!" You might find yourself being dragged into the thought, but there will be a moment where you will say to yourself, "Hang on! I was doing a walking meditation." Then you 'thank' the thought for sharing and continue with the exercise in the present moment.

You don't have to walk to be in a mindful meditation. You could be making a cup of tea, or ironing a shirt, or making a bed. The way of removing thought is by bringing your attention totally to the present action that you are undertaking.

Making the tea, you walk to the kettle, you extend your arm, your hand opens, and your fingers close around the handle. You lift the kettle from its base, feel its weight in your hand, and your body as it turns slowly toward the source of water. And so it continues, moment by moment. Give it a go. Try for one minute with a mindful meditation, then five, then ten etc.

You can also do this sitting or standing still or moving around. If sitting, you could start with your toes, feeling them move, maybe inside your shoes. Feeling the texture of your socks, or the inside surface of the shoe. Moving your ankles and feeling the joints flex. Bringing your attention up your legs and feeling the consistency of whatever you are sitting on, be it a cushioned seat or a wooden chair, stretching up through your spine and into your neck, gently moving your head and feeling the elasticity of your neck muscles. As thoughts try to enter, recognize their presence, and then let them go. Bring your attention back to the present exercise. The time between realizing that a thought has intruded and you have become lost in it will reduce with practice. Practice makes perfect, don't you know!

Again, I 'knew' this, yet the constant bombardment of fearful thoughts can persist, like, "Is my mother going to die before I get to her?", like my brother did. And angry thoughts, like, "Where is her support system over there?"

Over that next month in London caring for my mother, I lost weight. I knew it was happening, but I also knew why it was happening and it was *nothing* to do with the name of a disease. I was allowing the stress of the moment to affect me on a deeper physical level. Because I had these tools, I was able to bring myself back, without things getting to the past high levels of bowel inflammation or any ulceration, or bleeding etc. I didn't need any drugs.

I am not saying, "Do not take drugs or medication." Sometimes we need some support through the hard times, or if we haven't yet got a good handle on 'acceptance'. Everything has a place in this world, I guess, even though much of it seems madness at times!

So here I was in London, only 14 days after I was there last. As soon as I had dropped my bags at Barons Court, I went into the hospital to see my mother and I was shocked. When I'd last seen her, just two weeks earlier, Mum would have been ten kilos heavier. She has never been overweight and a loss of ten kilos was a lot for her.

I held myself together and donned my pragmatic hat – that is, what is the 'what is' and what can be done right now? The 'what is', was that they, the hospital staff, were not having any success in finding the right antibiotic to kill the aggressive bug affecting her. There were keeping her hydrated with a saline solution, but not with any nutrition. Much like any government-funded facility, the NHS struggled with too many patients and not enough beds or attending staff. The nurses were always 'rushed off their feet'. When meals arrived for my mother, they were plonked down on her bed table and left. Because my mother was now so weak, she spent a lot of the time sleeping. When she awoke, her food was cold. Her weakness made her hands shake, so even trying to get the food from the plate to her mouth was a huge effort and the experience of the cold hospital food was enough to discontinue eating.

I got her on nasal feeding straight away.

With the lack of food, a lack of energy had taken over her. With the constant diarrhea and vomiting that the bug caused, the will to live was leaving her.

But through all of this suffering, I have never seen my mother so beautiful – so present, so accepting, and so in the moment – she seemed to just glow. That is the only way I can describe it. In between her brief moments of tears of frustration with what was going on with her body and her inability to control it, as we sat together, sharing this time, she would just smile, constantly, almost like she was finally relaxing into a place of acceptance. Her skin was like alabaster and her eyes so blue; so beautiful, so peaceful.

She told me that she had had enough. I accepted this. I told her that if she wanted to go, that was fine. I shared that if I were suffering in the way that she was suffering, I would want to go too.

But, I told her that if she wanted to stay, she had to be on my team. I said this quite firmly.

She turned her head and looked up at me and quietly whispered, "I want to be on your team."

Tears welled up in my eyes and I asked her to repeat what she said, but louder. And in a stronger voice, she repeated, "I want to be on your team!"

Right! That was it. This was happening, I was going to make it happen.

Every day for a month, I walked across that graveyard from her house in Barons Court, to the Charing Cross Hospital, a hospital I had spent many a month in each year during my younger years.

I brought my mother her favorite foods, for breakfast, lunch, and dinner. Breakfast would be scrambled eggs and crispy, crispy bacon, just as she liked it. Lunch and dinner always included something she especially liked, as I needed to get her stimulated and enthused to eat again, even though shortly after she ate, it would all be expelled.

Funnily enough, I never experienced revulsion. I was surprised at myself by this, as I held her hands on one end of her, while a nurse cleaned her up on the other. I didn't really see or smell anything that caused me to gag, yet my mother was always so apologetic and felt so bad about what was happening to her in front of me. I told her that all I could see was her and nothing else.

I downloaded old Irish songs I knew she would know from the internet and sang them to her while she drifted in and out of consciousness. The best thing was seeing a small smile of recognition on her lips grow whilst hearing me sing with her eyes still closed.

I did things that I never, ever thought I would do, like wash and massage my mother's feet, clean and moisturize her face and hands, brush her hair and stroke her head. My aim was to nurture her to wellness, I guess, but I really wasn't doing anything with planned thought, it all just happened naturally.

Then finally, 'they', the doctors found an antibiotic that her body accepted. Major relief! The turnaround was finally happening and Mum was on her way back to life.

And here was the amusing part. As she got better, that smiling glow of acceptance wasn't always there! Her old behavior patterns started to return, subtly at first and then at times a little more obviously. Her non-acceptance was back, although I did help her recognize those moments and remind her that her 'no's' were only going to make her suffer! Sometimes she would smile in recognition, and at other times, she would just dismiss me! She was definitely getting better health-wise! How ironic.

I do remember my mother once telling me that when I was sick, I was a much nicer person! I'm not sure that it was so much because I was nicer, perhaps more that I needed her. Now I can understand that she preferred it when I needed her help, as opposed to when I didn't. This fed her co-dependency, her need to be needed, which many of us feel from time to time. It's probably how a favorite toy might feel – if it could – when a child discards it after many early years of total attachment. Or like when you make a friend and that friend attaches him or herself to you, to learn or gain as much as they can. Then once they can stand on their own two feet, or feel that they have sufficiently taken from you all that they need, they then might discard you too, much like the toy.

With my father's 'dysfunctional actions' and my mother's acceptance of them, I learnt to be a 'people pleaser' too. That term now turns my stomach! The funny thing here is that my life, if observed by an outsider, continually involves the energy of 'helping' people, and I could still be seen as a people pleaser. However, there's a distinct difference, which keeps me free.

I no longer please others to please myself. I just share with what I have within me. And there is no limited supply, because, ultimately, it's just 'energy'. I also no longer have any attachment to the outcome, so if someone has no affinity or understanding of what I'm sharing, that's okay now!

Do you remember the exhausting times you may have had trying to make someone understand the point you are telling him or her? Do you remember the feeling of anger in the pit of your stomach when they don't 'get' it and even worse, argue the point with you? The attachment to being 'right' for humans is massive, as I have mentioned before. I'm guessing that this is because if someone is trying to make us be in the wrong, then our whole identity is being challenged. And what are we taught to do when we are challenged? Fight back of course!

So back to Mum and her battle. It took one whole month, every day, pretty much, being at the hospital. By the end of that time, she had put on weight and had color in her cheeks. It was awesome to see.

Yes, finding the right antibiotic to kill the bug definitely stopped the attack on her body, but her decision to hang around a bit more – to be 'on my team' – was the driving force behind her recovery.

She shared with me a dream she had when I first arrived at the hospital, which gave her a choice between two directions. One of those choices was me, apparently, on top of a mountain. And she chose to take that direction. Her mind was made up, and her body followed.

There is increasing mention of the effects of the brain on the body in the media, documentaries, and books, which is so good. If I had attempted to write this book ten, twenty, or thirty years ago, its contents would have been hard to accept by many.

My time during the month of my mother's illness, did affect my body. I have already mentioned that I lost weight during this period. However, it was not so much due to the worry that I allowed to cross my mind, but more to do with the fact that I seemed to have less of an appetite for food. My attention was elsewhere, and eating was a backseat requirement. But what I *did* notice was that the pains were not there this time. The situation was a high level of stress, especially in the early part of that month when it appeared very likely that my mother would die and I was getting very little family support. I knew that I was going to have to accept the 'what is', whatever the 'what is' was going to be, in every moment that came, so I didn't concentrate on the 'what should be' and stress didn't cloud my mind.

Mum was fully recovered by the end of July. She came out of hospital, and I went back to Australia. Life went on.

Chapter 9

The Path to Self Discovery

In 2010, I returned to my house in Tasmania. The house, although beautiful, needed some large helpings of tender loving care, especially the West wall, as that got the brunt of the rough weather from, you guessed it, the West! The cedar wall needed replacing and the house needed painting. I had to make a decision as to whether I was going to sell the place or rent it out again.

I had bought this property seven years ago, a beautiful piece of sky, yet I could not afford to live in it, as there was no work for me in the Central Coast of Tasmania. So I had the house rented out. Every penny I made went to my huge mortgages. Since having breast cancer, I had sold off two other properties to cut down my debts, as owning property was becoming less attractive to me. Unfortunately, being a self-employed make-up artist and photographer, living from job to job and always traveling – debt always had a funny way of creeping up again! So as I hadn't lived in the house, I thought I might as well just cut my losses and be free from those heavy chains of debt.

I got a couple of quotes amounting to around $20,000 – which I didn't have – and, as a bit of a do-it-yourselfer, I entertained the idea of managing the project myself and beating that budget!

What to do? Well, in the end, I decided to drive to Tasmania myself, organize two friends, my long-time carpenter friend, Matt, and my beautiful electrician friend, Beau, to come over and do some paid work on the house. It was an amazing experience, which started with my solo trip down to Tasmania in my Ford Falcon wagon, packed to the roof with camping equipment to survive in a big empty house over this time.

The plan in the beginning was to fix the house up and sell it. Don't you love plans? The Yiddish saying, "Man plans and God laughs" is so true! With all the plans we make, you can *never* guarantee that they will work out exactly the way you thought they would. If you have an attachment that they should, and they don't, well, welcome to suffering.

But something shifted in me once again, during these renovations. It was freezing cold – the Tasmanian winter is well set in by mid-June – and it rained a lot. I had the experience of how the wind can 'cut you to the bone', but the space, the trees, the birds, the sounds and then the total lack of them, in the sometimes deafening silence at night, all of it seemed to change something within me, quite like being cracked by an osteopath. Maybe more layers of my onion were being peeled away. Maybe, the peace of the nature all around me was 'speaking' or connecting with some part within myself – or the other way around. It was like the 'white noise' being switched off in my head. Just in case you are too young to remember, the white noise occurred when the television shut down for the night. After a band had played 'God Save The Queen', the screen would go white and speckled, and there would be this hissing noise. If you had fallen asleep during a movie, that's what you would wake up to, before you dragged yourself off to bed!

After a couple of weeks of extremely hard work and suffering cold and flu-like symptoms, I flew back to Brisbane to do two weeks of shooting. I then started the routine of flying back and forth to Tasmania, working on the house a little more by myself, camping in the house for two weeks and then flying up to Brisbane for work.

I moved between the green, spacious and quiet environment of a hilltop in Tasmania, to a more compact and noisy environment, right in the center of Brisbane. What is bizarre for me is that wherever I am now, I'm happy! I'm somewhat frustrated when my mind keeps trying to ask the question, "Well, where should I be?" The answer: exactly where I am.

I am a Caucasian female, living in the twenty-first century in a Western country. I am not a Buddhist monk, living around two and a half thousand years ago. Therefore, I have to adapt to the current existence of wherever I am, as I am, and act accordingly. Here, there's stuff – whether it be houses, cars, clothes, shoes, handbags, or whatever it is that we seem to surround ourselves with or escape into, for comfort or identification.

The most important thing for me to be aware of is the level at which I am attached to my 'things' and circumstances and how less and less this level of attachment is becoming. Observing these thoughts is both entertaining and enlightening and I watch myself and my thoughts now regularly.

I remember, as a Falun Dafa practitioner, selling my third motorbike, which I dearly loved. She was a Kawasaki 500S and red, therefore very fast! I frequently seemed to be unable to stick to the speed limit and therefore, at the time, felt I was attached to speed and adrenaline. With Buddhism, one is supposed to have no attachments, so I made the decision to sell the bike, just to see if I could. I put an ad in the paper and, straightaway, I had interest. The first lady that came along loved her. The next thing I knew, I had cash in my pocket and I was waving her goodbye. It was at least two hours before I realized that I had sold the bike and she was gone! And I hadn't been *that* moved. Now some might say here that I obviously didn't love the bike enough. Not true. I loved riding that particular bike, she was so easy to maneuver and had great acceleration!

The point I'm wishing to make here is that everything and every person in this life is temporary. So perhaps if we could 'see' that all is on loan, then maybe we might respect and enjoy everything more, as we never know when change is going to come along and a treasured person, or item is lost to us. Perhaps, if we concentrated more on being true to our essential nature – you know, that space between all our molecules – and practiced more unconditional and unattached love to all beings and all things, then we would experience so much more freedom for ourselves and lessen not only our suffering in this world but also others.

This path of self-discovery and enlightenment is sometimes a very lonely one. Most of the time, one is surrounded by others that see this world as 'real' and love the 'attachments' that they have.

When one gets to see through the veil as such, and see life in a different way, one's path can become very solitary, with not many like-minded people walking alongside you, so you end up keeping quiet about your deepest thoughts. I know I do. To find others, who resonate in the same way as yourself, is a rarity and a blessing when you meet them.

Rama Krishna said:

> When you first begin to awaken, you are like a tiny little tree. It is good to surround this small tree with a fence, so it does not get stepped upon by the cows. Later, when the tree gets big and strong, it can give shade to many, many people, but at first it's really good to have it protected.

I guess this is what happened for me in 2000. I came across a group of like-minded people when I had my first major shift of thinking, others that shared my values and feelings and reassured me that I hadn't gone completely crazy, which most of my other friends thought I had.

Again, once you get a taste for this type of truth, it's almost impossible to go back. I found that who I thought I was, what I was doing, no longer fitted into this present mindset. I had to keep letting go of it though, as my mind kept bringing in previous mindsets, past ways of thinking and being. This practice of constant observation of my mind and, in turn, my behavior, allows me to continually move onto new levels of understanding.

I write a lot, as I have already mentioned. I write down anything that comes to mind in the moment, and on anything that I have to hand, or now record on my phone. In the past, some dear friends gave me beautiful notebooks and I write my thoughts and understandings in them as they come to me – especially the ones that pop into my head in the early hours of the morning and wake me up. There is always a notebook and a pen beside me where I sleep, wherever that is.

Just now, there is a page open in one of my notebooks on my desk here, dated 30 January 2009.

> Your mind will prevent you from understanding
> And your eyes will prevent you from 'seeing'
> But your heart will always have the ability to see and recognize the Truth.

Now, part of your mind could still be sitting with those old 'I knows' and this may cause you to judge my thoughts. Just remember, whenever we judge something, it never determines the person or the thing we judge, it simply means that we are someone who judges.

It really doesn't matter what you believe, or perceive, but one thing is blindingly obvious. There is more than we presently know. If there weren't, how could we keep learning new things? And if there is 'more', how can we ever be so ignorant or so arrogant, for that matter, as to think it can only be this way or that? Surely, if whatever works, works, then that's the 'what is'. Isn't it?

I have no attachment any more that another should understand me and that gives me so much peace. My mother at times would say that I don't care, but that's not it at all. That's just her negative perception. It is not that I don't care how another thinks; it is that I now totally accept another's perception, especially when it differs from mine. This is so far from how I used to think!

I cannot control anything outside myself – how you think, how my mother or another family member thinks, what anyone thinks. I can only choose how to use my thoughts and what I have within myself. How I choose to use this energy will determine the next part of my journey.

I still have questions and the most prevalent ones are always, "What am I supposed to do next? Where am I supposed to be next?" It takes just a few moments and then I can smile at myself. Because with the practice of acceptance of each present moment, I can be happy with being exactly where I am and doing exactly what I'm doing. And right now, that is me sharing with you!

This almost seems like a letter to a dear friend for whom I want the best. And that is *so* true. I admit that it is a very long letter; yet, there is still so much more to impart. As I said in the very beginning, the message I want to convey to you, to give you freedom from whatever suffering you are experiencing, is simple. To repeat it once again: it is acceptance. Acceptance with love: this, and this alone, will give you the clarity you need for your next action.

Here's a beautiful story I heard while listening to a lecture by Ram Dass, which outlines how acceptance works so well with life here.

Once there was a farmer who had a horse, but the horse ran away. The neighbor said to the farmer, "Oh, isn't that too bad!" And the farmer said, "You never know." The next day, the horse came back followed by a beautiful wild stallion. And the neighbor said, "How fortunate!" and the farmer said, "You never know." And shortly thereafter, the son of the farmer was riding the wild stallion and he fell and broke his leg. And the neighbor said, "Isn't that terrible?" and the farmer said, "You never know." Shortly after that, government officials were coming through the village, conscripting the young men for service. Because the boy had a broken leg, he was left behind. And the neighbor said, "How fortunate!" And the farmer said, "You never know."

Apply this way of being through life and you will experience less stress.

I haven't meant to create a mini-autobiography; however, it can help us to understand where we are by showing where we have been.

My intention is to show you my path and hope that it enlightens you to the fact that no matter where you have been, no matter what has or has not been 'done' to you, you still have the ability to fundamentally change your life right now. It all starts with the mind and the taught or pre-conditioned way of thinking. Therefore, it must change with the mind and a different way of thinking.

It seems that we come here, devoid of personal gain, just survival techniques, and then we get taught that the world has to give us what we want. And when we don't get what we want, or we don't like what we get, we react to that with non-acceptance. Reactions and those thoughts of "No!" are the 'things' that destroy us from the inside out.

"No matter how big, or how small, whatever bond holds you, release yourself from it. With each release, the closer you will come to where you are meant to be next." That's another of my little messages to myself.

Keep hold of your 'truth', it will always be there, yet 'life' has a way of blurring the lines and sometimes it gets buried and forgotten.

No matter what you have absorbed from the moments in your life and what you have made them mean, know that you are solely responsible for what you are making them mean right here and right now. Know that you are the one sending yourself messages throughout your life, your stories. Don't concern yourself anymore with where you learnt them. That is the past. The question is, where is the truth in your story right here in the 'now'?

If the story you come up with about something, such as a task you are about to do, is, "It's too hard", then you will give up on the task, or do it half-heartedly, because of the 'story' you have in the back of your mind. But what if you change the message that you are sending yourself? What if you change the story to, "It's easy and enjoyable!"?

Until the task is done, the reality of whether the task was easy or difficult to complete does not exist. By using the story of the task being, "It's easy" as opposed to "It's too hard", the task will be perceived by you from an 'easy' angle and therefore have more of a chance of being just that.

I remember once complaining to a friend of mine that I had to go and do a make-up and hair job at a glamor studio the following day. I moaned that the money was terrible, the conversations would be boring and the day would just seem so long! She suggested that I changed the way I thought about the job. So the following morning, on my way to this job, I reminded myself that I was going to have a fabulous day, that I was being paid the equivalent of a million dollars and the people I would meet would be amazing and we would have awesome conversations and the day would breeze by! And it worked! I had the best day ever!

So apply this to your life. Start to change all the negative 'messages' that you are sending yourself and exchange them for positive messages – that is, yes, I'm mentioning this again, unless you enjoy suffering. It comes with practice and you need to observe your mind on a constant basis, or it will definitely fall back to old behavior patterns.

I spoke with a woman not long ago at a friend's social gathering. Her daughter had been diagnosed with Crohn's disease, but was currently in 'remission', which obviously means that she believed her daughter still had the disease, but that it's just 'sleeping' for the moment.

When I shared my understanding with her that I don't have Crohn's disease, her first question was, "How did you get rid of 'It'?"

When I explained to her that to me, 'It' is nothing more than a name for symptoms that are currently being experienced in the body, her attachment to her 'I knows' came straight to the fore. "Of course there's an '*It*'!" she exclaimed, "My daughter only has to get stressed about exams or something and *It* flares up again!"

I told her that I accepted that she understood it in this way. However, I wanted to share with her another understanding. But her body language indicated that her need to hold on to what she already knew was too strong and I recognized that I had to just let it go. When she said that her daughter had to avoid stress, as it aggravated her Crohn's disease, I would have liked to suggest that it was the daughter's stressful thoughts that caused the inflammation in the bowel, as previously explained. We were interrupted just at that point and her attention turned to the new arrival. Our conversation had been terminated. I observed myself, happy in the knowledge that I didn't have to make her wrong and myself right.

I remember once speaking with a new doctor, who was checking me for moles on my skin, follow ups after the removal of my malignant mole, previously shared.

While looking at my medical file, she noticed that I had been previously diagnosed with Crohn's disease. "Ah!" she said, "How are you going with your Crohn's?" I started to explain to her that I no longer had Crohn's disease and that I was going fine. Her medical mind kicked in and she informed me that I was obviously managing my Crohn's well, as there was no 'cure' for Crohn's disease.

Well, seeing as there is no definite explanation for what causes Crohn's disease in the medical world, how could they accept that there is a cure for it? 'It' doesn't exist! It's just a name!

'*It*' is just a name that has been given to the inflammation and ulceration of tissue in the gastrointestinal tract. So, without the name, it is just inflammation and ulceration. So, without the inflammation and ulceration, what is '*It*' now? Nothing!

This is not like the eternal question of the chicken and the egg! The inflammation and consequent ulceration are symptoms, brought on by a 'cause'. The cause is what should be looked at.

Wayne Dyer once said, "An ulcer is the result of a chemical change in the body, brought on by thinking." So glad more minds out there are being enlightened to this!

The most important thing is to let go of the ownership of a name, or your mind will hold on to it and it will become part of your identity, thereby giving 'It' the opportunity to exist.

So now change your story from, "I have Crohn's disease" to "I am currently experiencing the physical symptoms of..." and "I accept that this is what is happening in my body right here and right now" *and* "I also accept that this is a result of an external situation that my mind is responding to and, in turn, affecting my body."

A good book to read by Rick Hanson PhD with Richard Mendius MD is *Buddha's Brain: The Practical Neuroscience of Happiness, Love, and Wisdom*, where you can find practical exercises to stimulate and strengthen your brain, which will in turn make it easier to 'choose' the positive thoughts and let go of the negative ones.

There are many different ways that you can be free from a destructive mind pattern, and seeking out a way of doing this is one of the most important things that you should be doing while you are on this planet!

When you are free from your destructive or negative thoughts, your life becomes less encumbered. You will no longer be self-destructive when 'bad' or 'negative' things happen in your life, because through learning acceptance of every moment, you will have the peace and clarity within you to be able to act – again, accepting the 'what is' and taking the moment that has happened and forming the next one with a positive mindset.

The work of another philosopher, psychiatrist and physician I have studied is Dr. David Hawkins. He describes a 'Map of Consciousness' and talks about the level of energy that is held within each emotion. The logic is obvious, but perhaps easily dismissed by an academic, unless they have an understanding and acceptance of kinesiology. In this map, Dr. Hawkins talks about the emotions that range from enlightenment right through to shame, individually naming and quantifying seventeen emotions. He suggests that having a view of life with peace, for instance, is a high level of energy, constantly giving back to the individual that embraces it. In contrast, shame is at a very low level of energy, which depletes.

To summarize in my words, any negative emotion that you hold within you drains you of energy with its destructive power. Any positive emotion that you hold within you elevates you with energy and creates constructive power. How metaphorically heavy does an individual feel when depressed? And how light does an individual feel when happy?

You may think that you do not have a choice about how you feel. You may wish to believe that everything outside of yourself contributes to your emotions. To a degree, it does – but only when you place meaning upon it.

Here you are in a happy mood in the supermarket. You have money in your pocket and you are shopping for ingredients to make a surprise meal for someone special. As you are moving around the aisles, you move lightly. You are happy! As you finish shopping, you make your way to the check out, looking forward to the delicious outcome of your purchases. Just as you approach the queue, someone pushes their trolley in front of yours, hitting it as they go. Please meet the Angry Trolley Pusher (ATP). I may have mentioned him or her already! Before you have a chance to speak, the Angry Trolley Pusher starts barking at you and actually blames you for running into their trolley!

And now, in this moment, here is your choice: acceptance and then action, or, non-acceptance and reaction.

What are you going to make this episode mean? What is the 'truth' of this moment?

The truth is, here is an ATP. For whatever reason, this person is angry. What you make their behavior mean to you is your business. But be warned, you will be personalizing the episode. This is not reality. You are not here to change others. You are here to change yourself. By changing yourself and freeing yourself from suffering, *then* you can help others.

In the past, my first reaction to the ATP would have been to reciprocate that anger. How dare this person invalidate my existence and push in front of me! And worse, *dare* to hit my trolley! And worse still, dare to attack *me*!

This is obviously an example of non-acceptance in action and my ego coming through! This could then escalate the negative energy, by me making some comment to this already Angry Trolley Pusher. That would only add fuel to the fire, exactly what they were seeking in the first place! This scenario has the probability of only becoming worse.

At the same time that you are reacting to this angry person with your own anger, your blood is rushing to your gut area, getting ready for fight or flight. This in turn is placing the white blood cells in an area ready for invasion and ready to counter attack. There is more to come shortly on this topic, as when Dr. Bruce Lipton's work was recently introduced to me, more light was thrown onto this subject.

Back to the supermarket!

So say you choose acceptance. The 'what is' is that here is an angry person. You don't know what their life is like, what they go through etc. The only 'known' fact is what you know yourself. Don't use past experiences and let your ego jump up and down for you in self-protection mode. Don't make the situation personal. This angry person is looking for situations to satisfy their anger. Becoming angry too is exactly what they are looking for! They are like walking upsets waiting to happen, much like Trolls on the internet. How exhausting for them!

Again, my first action is to immediately apologize! I know, it sounds crazy, but it usually works like a dream. I follow the apology with an honest smile (no, not a sarcastic one, that would be a past behavior!) The ATP is now stumped. Usually, when the ATP behaves in this way, the 'victim' would normally fight back, feeding the ATP's need for anger and aggression.

If you don't pick up the racquet, the game cannot continue. You don't need to become another ATP. You need to be authentic to yourself, remember? Peace, joy and love and so on.

I have already discussed the effect anger has on the body, so why would you allow some crazy ATP to change your peaceful and happy shopping state and cause you to self-damage?

The ATP is angry and looking for an opportunity to get upset. That's the 'what is'. Therefore, their action of pushing in has absolutely nothing to do with you. So, logic begs that you do NOT allow yourself to change from your happy state into one of anger and revenge!

Whatever is inside the person comes out.

As previously discussed, the moment you were born, (from a peaceful pregnancy) you had no knowledge or experience of your own emotions. You were hopefully pure joy, wonderment, and love. This I see as you in your most authentic state.

As experiences of life are introduced to you, some negative emotions are learnt along the way. It's like the injected orange.

So, if you ever hear an angry word from someone to yourself, this is only coming from him or her, due to their own mental suffering. It has nothing to do with you. You are just a convenient target for them to expel the bad feeling that they have inside of them. They don't seem to understand how to get rid of it any other way, other than to make another as miserable as they are and then be reaffirmed with their self-created identity, when you hit back at them, returning the serve. This is only how they perceive their life should be, because that's what it has been in the past. This is what they have been taught. This is what I was taught.

It is so sad, because it is it's so simple to be another way – simple, but not always easy.

Chapter 10

The Choices We Make

So, now you know. It's all about choice, and knowing that you have a choice. If you do feel 'bad', know that you are choosing to feel so. I am guessing some of you won't like that sentence. I know I wouldn't have in the past. Why would I *choose* to feel bad! But that is exactly what is going on. Something 'bad' happens and the only way we can avoid suffering as a result, is to step back and choose how we are going to feel about the 'happening'. Sometimes this is a hard thing to do, especially if you have been taught by others to externalize your pain and look outside yourself to blame the source of your 'feeling bad' as I was. Blaming externally was a far easier option.

By stepping back and finding that space, there you will find the ability to accept and then act. "Surely, backing down when someone attacks you is just being weak?" I hear you say. Well, it's actually much harder to step back. A reflex is something that happens without conscious thought which is useful at times but mostly destructive at others. To find the space, to step back to consider and accept, that's the strength.

I feel that you are here to live and experience your own life. If there's anything that is not working for you, fix that first and then you can help others – not by telling them that they are wrong, but by 'being' who you want to be. This is how you change the behavior of others around you.

We learn by observation. Often, a couple can be so used to arguing, that they see it as an affectionate way of 'being' towards each other. Yet, the nasty words said, or negative actions deployed, even under the guise of jest, creep in and cause resentment at an subconscious level. This then builds up and can result in larger and more volatile arguments and unhappy relationships, or even terminated ones.

Meanwhile, if any children are in the vicinity of this energy, then this is all passed on to them as tools for them to behave with. This is where the illusion that we all become trapped in begins.

Our lives are ruled by our beliefs. Our beliefs are created by our own personal and individual understanding of the judgments that we make about a certain situation. This is our perception. So, our perceptions become our beliefs. We base our stories on our beliefs and this becomes the way we run our lives. Not much reality here at all! We just perceive, then judge! And how we were first taught to perceive determines how we will continue.

Can you believe this? All these beings walking around on this planet with all these different perceptions, stories, and beliefs! No wonder it's crazy here at times!

So how do we change it all? Understanding what perception is could be a place to start.

Learning, Memory and Expectation

Perception is the process of attaining awareness or understanding of the environment, by organizing and interpreting sensory information. All perception involves signals in the nervous system, which in turn result from physical stimulation of the sense organs. Vision involves light striking the retinas of the eyes, smell is the awareness of odor molecules, and hearing involves pressure waves. Perception is not the passive receipt of these signals, but can be shaped by *learning, memory, and expectation.*

And then here's the 'kicker'. Perception depends on these functions of the nervous system, but *subjectively* seems most effortless because this processing *happens outside of conscious awareness.*

Considering everything is made up of molecules, with different densities, different structures, then adding to this, all these people running around this planet with their own perceptions of this molecular muddle, one would be right to say that this is a 'mad, mad world'!

So, now having an understanding of perception, now knowing that we are walking around 'seeing' the world through glasses with different prescriptions, you just have to decide here as to how you want your life to be.

You need to sit back and work out what messages you are sending yourself, all of which you have learnt from past experiences and adding to this, your individual perception of those past experiences. Is whatever you are doing or thinking presently working for you? Are you suffering? If so, how are you suffering?

Now the problem here, of course, is that with every question you have, the way that you presently use your mind is how you are going to come up with an answer! Hmmm... not safe really, considering that your perception could still be a little out of whack!

To illustrate how even a very brief moment of trauma can have a lasting impact on your mind, the psychological kinesiologist, Rob Williams MA, who uses kinesiology to 'rewire' the brain, tells a story about a little girl.

She was traveling in a car with her family across the Eastern Plains of Colorado having, what she perceived as 'fun', in the back seat, which was seen as misbehavior by her mother. At her young age, she was just bored with the long drive and wanted attention.

The parents were hot and bothered, the drive had been long and their patience was wearing thin. The mother barked at her daughter and told her to behave, or she would stop the car and leave her behind. Of course, the little girl didn't believe her (she hadn't experienced abandonment, obviously) and continued her self-amusement by kicking the back of the drivers seat. The car was violently pulled over. The mother got out of the car and walking around to the other side of the car, opened the back door and silently pulled the little girl out of her seat. She then closed the door, walked back around to the driver's seat and drove off. The car came back within minutes of its departure, but in that time, the little girl's perception of wide-open spaces became associated with fear, anxiety and panic.

Now this is probably something that many parents have warned and even done to their children in the past, as a form of control. But perhaps being left in the middle of the desert plains is a bit of an extreme location to learn this particular lesson!

Shortly after this episode, she displayed fear of and anxiety about going out of her house. For the next 56 years of her life, she was an agoraphobic, having fear of open spaces, which ruled her life. She came across Rob Williams, who used the practice of kinesiology with her, which fundamentally changed her way, her perception, of seeing wide, open spaces. She was then able to go outside freely, learn to drive a car and be independent. Apparently, this all changed for her in just one session. Clinical hypnotherapy is another effective technique used to achieve changes in the way that we think.

I would love to be able to say to you that there is only one way for you to change your perceptions, but this is definitely not the case. These changes can be dramatic and very quick. Just because it took 'x' number of years to get you to here, it can sometimes only take you a few minutes to get you out of this place! You also don't necessarily have to plough through every event that's ever happened in your life in order to free yourself from it. It's being aware in the moment that a message your mind might be sending you right now is negative. It's about being present, right here right now, and deciding for yourself as to whether or not you will 'choose' this thought and let it hang around any longer.

For the lady who suffered agoraphobia for 56 years, kinesiology was the key. For me, suffering with this named Crohn's disease for 40 years, it was reading and absorbing words in a book of Buddhist lectures.

You may feel that your thinking might be so set and strong, that all the words that could be read or listened to would not create change within you at all. But I don't really believe that. I believe that anyone can change their life, no matter what they have done in the past, or how they presently think. Again, here I am as a white crow. I had 40 years of 'programming' and was re-booted within seven days! Less than! Some people 'wake up' even faster than that.

And there's another key point. You might have heard the saying, "Oh, he won't change until he's ready to change." Absolutely. Everyone is on his or her own path here and different things will affect people in different ways, depending on their current way of thinking. You need to want the change. Change usually comes about when we are ready or desperate for it. It can come with just one word, one sentence or from a fifteen-second-life experience. Chaos or a catastrophic event may bring it about. Personal suffering that comes to a peak may cause you to finally choose to make a change in your life. Whatever it is, or isn't, just know that your life is the way that it is as a result of your choices and if you don't like what is happening, *choose something else!* Choose change!

In the Bible it is written that Jesus said, "Why do you look at the speck that is in your brother's eye, but do not notice the log that is in your own eye?" (Matthew 7:3) This may be another way of saying, 'Look within yourself. Consider that what you think you see in another, may be a small mirror of a larger problem you have yourself'. Make sure you clear up your own mind/heart, before looking at another. You will see more 'truth' this way and in turn, you can help others in a better way. If we all did this, cleared ourselves right up, and then had the desire to help and free others, what an amazing world this could be!

My mind created the dis-ease in my body and the release of my past way of thinking, allowed my body to heal itself. Please, just give it a go.

As I mentioned earlier, I now practice standing 'nowhere', as it's the safest place I've found to be. I've heard another saying which mirrors this. "Stand midway between hope and hopelessness." Beautiful.

With no attachment to any outcomes, just with the acceptance of 'what is'; it is here you will find the peace you've been searching for.

When I am presented with something in the moment, I like to check it out to see why it came across my path. I came across Dr. Bruce Lipton's work in *The Biology of Belief* after I had completed the main bulk of my book. I watched a YouTube video clip of one of his lectures and was blown away by how his scientific and biological knowledge explained everything that I had done in getting rid of Crohn's disease. It all made such perfect sense! It was so excellent to see and hear scientific facts explain my unscientific thinking, everything that I have been through in my life, what I have done with what I've learnt and then achieved with my present health and wellbeing! I was so impressed with Dr. Lipton's work, so much so that I had to rewrite this book to mention his work in it!

For those of you with academic or scientific minds, I urge you to investigate the actual workings of cells in the body. When you do, you will find that it is the environment that has an affect on the cell. What does this mean? Fear for some of you, no doubt, because you will now *have* to take responsibility for how you run this ship from now on. The old way of thinking, Newtonian physics, which had a belief system of matter, kept people thinking that genes controlled 'life'. This is no longer true. You can remove the genes from a cell and the cell still functions. Life is the *movement* of the proteins in the cells. Wow!

In 1925, quantum physics brought in the understanding that 'the universe is based on energy, not matter'. However, even now, conventional medicine still bases its science on matter and has not really brought in the nature of quantum physics and, in turn, is therefore no longer science.

The reason? Conventional medicine still insists on working on a material system in order to provide matter problems with matter solutions! Yes, you've guessed it! Problems = illness, and solutions = drugs.

Not too long ago, there was a move to stop placebo testing alongside new medication testing! Now why would they want to do that? My thoughts? If the placebo tests have the same, or close to the same results as the chemical tests, as previously discussed, this rather invalidates the chemical medications as a preferred solution, doesn't it? Placebos, as I've mentioned before, are being shown to have very similar success rates, without the harmful side effects, unlike chemical medications. So where does that leave the pharmaceutical companies and their profits? At a loss.

Also, more control is being exercised on the 'alternative healthcare industry'. They, *they* being the pharmaceutical chaps who are desperate for control over this industry, have been trying for years to harness the natural therapy products, to ban anything that hasn't been tested and 'something, something' approved!

The way I see it is, if it really is 95% of us who can alter our cell behavior by changing the signals we send them, then surely we should take the responsibility back– the power back, if you like – to ourselves.

So how do we work out what is a 'curable' disease and how can it be overcome and changed by the way that we think, to what is an 'incurable' disease, the ones which need medication, medical treatment, and operations and so on?

Dr. Lipton explains this well in *The Biology of Belief.* He introduces the understanding that it is the signals that affect the proteins in the cells that produces the characteristics of life.

What is responsible for the alterations of behavior or the state of a dis-ease? What can that be attributed to? Lipton's answer: proteins or signals.

Another question he raised was how much of our dis-eased states might be related to the protein and how much might be related to the signals that activate the proteins?

His understanding is that less than 5% of a population can actually claim that their lives are affected by not having the appropriate proteins. These people were born with alterations in the DNA, called mutations or birth defects, which led to the production of a protein that does not work properly.

So, with this understanding that so few of the population can legitimately claim that their biology is affected by defective proteins, that then leaves us with a question about the other 95% or so of the population. When they get sick, when they get a disease, what can the problem be attributed to in their case?

It can't be the proteins, as they were already installed with an intact genome and therefore have the ability to create all the normal proteins. So, if it's not the proteins that are causing the defects, there's only one other component to the action! It's the signal! Dr. Lipton explains that this can happen in three ways. It can happen through trauma, which can distort the message and the signal to the cell causing disease, chemical and poisons being introduced into the body or inappropriate activating behavior/signals.

I could continue quoting Lipton's work, but this is your journey and you need to do your own discovering. I find his work fascinating, especially as it helps me understand how my journey has been so effective!

I would like to add my thoughts on the environments in which cells can be affected:

- The 'energy' within our home and work life, feeling happy or unhappy.

- The food we eat and the liquids we drink, as well as how we are 'feeling' whilst we eat. What we inhale or inject and medicines we take.

- The exposure to bacterial, viral or chemical elements, toxins, or poisons introduced via insect or animal bites.

- The environment between our ears, the subconscious mind. This I believe to be the major one!

Considering the speed and process of information that the subconscious mind can handle, in contrast to what the conscious mind can handle, keeping an eye on the conscious mind at *all times* is hard or, perhaps one could say, almost impossible!

Our subconscious mind operates all regions of the brain. It is a database for all our habitual and learnt perceptions. These then become stored (as stories) and require no processing – i.e. no thought.

Perceptions are how we 'read' a situation in our environment. These become automatic and habitual, due to repetition and then become built into the subconscious mind.

The conscious mind runs in live time. It is the creative mind, associated with the 'identity' of self and spiritual self.

Dr Bruce Lipton mentions the driving lesson in *The Biology of Belief* as an example of the two separate consciousnesses. I love it! He explains that if you were learning to drive a car, your conscious mind is very present, trying to absorb all these different bits of information, concentrating on the motion of all actions required to perform the task at hand. Once the mechanisms are learnt, these perceptions are now locked into the subconscious for driving. You now no longer have to be continually 'conscious' when driving a car! Scary huh? Your conscious thought might be, "I am going to drive to the shop for milk and bread." You get into your car and start it. You are off down the familiar road to the shop, with your subconscious mind driving and your conscious mind probably thinking about what else you might need at the shop! This highlights the fact that the subconscious mind can be operating without our conscious awareness!

So, if we have perceptions that are repeated continually, they then become locked into our subconscious mind and in turn, 'drive' our life. If the perceptions we hold are negative, we will definitely mismanage our own biology and not be aware at all that we are doing so!

There are so many different paths out there, to teach us better ways of living our lives and whatever works for you, is good. It is important for you to understand that there is a journey – that *this* is your journey, in which you can make changes to how you think and in turn how you feel.

If your life is fine as it is, then great, you may see no reason for change. However, if things aren't working out for you the way you would like, then change it!

A great quote I heard, by one of the many speakers I've listened to, came from a Russian philosopher, George Gurdjieff: "Were you to escape from prison, the first thing you must recognize is that you are in prison. If you think you are free, no escape is possible." Brilliant.

Chapter 11

Affirmation and Acceptance

You've heard of affirmations? Words and sentences constantly repeated until you believe them? Politicians use them all the time, so you end up believing them and vote them in! "Yes, we can!" "Yes, we can!" Sound familiar?

An affirmation is supposed to be a declaration of something that is true. However, an affirmation, or a 'self truth/belief', can be created by saying something over and over again, without containing any truth whatsoever.

So, if a parent tells a child continually that they are bad and stupid, is this true? No. The problem with this constant repetition is that it becomes an affirmation that the child then holds in their subconscious as a running 'story' and this in turn affects the way they see their world. Very often there is no separation seen by the parent between the behavior of the child and the child! How about telling the child that you love and accept the child, but that their behavior is not acceptable and will have consequences! This way, they can work out that they at least have a choice about how their day turns out! The other way leads to a path of self-destruction. Ask my brother when you see him.

So, we need to find out what old stories we have running in our subconscious, what we have programmed in it and what we now need to remove.

According to Louise Hay, "Every thought we think, every word we speak creates our future. If you change your thinking you can change your life." Many years ago, I remember reading her book *You Can Heal Your Life*, mentioned previously, when I started my search for something better than what I was currently experiencing with my bad health. I have not read the book since, but I think I remember reading something about removing the layers of an onion. These layers, in my understanding, are the perceptions that we cloak ourselves with, but in fact, they do not give us protection at all, but blind us from whom we really are.

Affirmations are the starting points for change. What really gives the affirmations power, is the energy put behind them, your intention and also your trust.

Brainwashing is the application of coercive techniques to change the values and beliefs, perceptions and judgments, and subsequent mindsets and behaviors of one or more people, usually for political, financial, personal, or religious purposes. How is this done? Coercive practices are not very nice, because they usually involve threats, intimidation, or other forms of pressure or force and they use the power of negative affirmations. But I think the key lesson here is understanding the effectiveness of affirmations alongside physical experience. A positive affirmation along with a positive physical experience is enough to change the subconscious. Finding out the best way of doing this for yourself, is part of your journey. There's no prescription for this, but one suggestion I have is investigating and trying out the Tapping Technique with Nic Ortner. Anthony Robbins has some great solutions too.

Whether your first step toward change is through religion or other belief systems, great. Just remember, that each religion, as with each belief system, has boundaries. In my understanding, boundaries, or laws of each particular system, prevents further change past those points. Use them all as stepping-stones along your journey.

Once the desire to change happens, doors start opening up all over the place! Once a path such as clinical hypnotherapy or kinesiology, or reading and listening to like-minded philosophers is commenced and keeping yourself present every step of the way, then you are definitely on your way to freedom.

I believe it is important to always be open for change. Eckhart Tolle puts it beautifully: "Be still enough to listen and be open enough to hear." If a person is so ruled by a particular thought process, and they bring their individual perception of that thought process into a present lesson of life, change will be hard to come by.

Now do you understand why it's important to drop your 'I knows'?

As is now obvious, an answer to a problem we may be having **cannot** be found outside of your Self. So, we need to turn within ourselves for the next answer and the possibility of change.

If you grasp the understanding that how you think creates your world, then you will know why your thinking is so important.

My thinking was programmed with repeated affirmations of:

You're stupid.

You're ugly.

You're worthless.

You don't deserve happiness.

You don't deserve financial freedom.

You won't amount to anything. You will fail at everything you attempt. You will never succeed.

You won't have any friends, but if you do, then they will just want you for what they can get from you.

And so on and so on.

So, no matter where these affirmations came from, once I recognized that they polluted my thinking, I needed to make a choice, to keep my running stories, or just drop them and replace them with new ones!

It's a no-brainer – however, only if you are open for change.

And, in 2000, I was. It seems that, when you are in that space of being still enough to listen and open enough to hear, a shift really can occur and sometimes a dramatic shift at that. Each experience is different for different people. You need to find the right experience to create your shift. So this is your journey. This is your path.

When you find it, not everyone else is going to be walking along the same path at the same pace. In fact – and I've touched on this already – sometimes this journey can seem very lonely. But then again, you are never lonely when you like the person you are alone with.

Ram Dass once mentioned that to find other similar souls walking in the same direction as you is sometimes hard and you are fortunate to find them. There are just so many people out there stuck in the exterior! Stuck in that old molecular muddle, placing so much importance on what they have 'without' and not concentrating and growing what they already have 'within'.

We need to come back to our center. Everything seems to point to something 'within'. Whatever you feel that 'within' is – the energy, the soul, the Christ consciousness, the Atman, whatever you refer to – all points to something 'within'.

It's Time To Make Up Your Mind

So now you know that you have a choice. You also know that in order to make a new choice for yourself, you have to fundamentally change the way your mind 'thinks'. You now understand that keeping your mind in the present moment will give you clarity. You also understand that the subconscious mind holds running stories, with access to all your experiences and other people's negative and positive affirmations of you.

How do you make the change? You make a 'conscious' decision, a 'present' choice; you tell yourself what messages you now want running in your mind or subconscious. Write them down if it helps. The rest will always be in there somewhere, but you are now 'choosing' to be more observant of your mind and keep the good messages running and let go of the bad ones. This library of the mind contains your beautiful memories; those that you want to keep and draw on from time to time. The ones you don't want or need anymore don't disappear from the shelves and may still pop up occasionally, but if you fundamentally change the way you think, your running story and the messages in your subconscious, then you will no longer be negatively affected by them. This way you will be practicing the 'power of now ' (thank you, Eckhart Tolle!) and observing your mind.

I am not going to claim that I have one specific answer for you that would personally change your life. I have just found the answer for me. By sharing my understandings with you and sharing the works of different people I have come across along my journey, perhaps this may help change the way you use your mind and improve your way of being.

As it has been said in some book somewhere, "Seek and ye shall find." I love that! That book, called the Bible, may have no facts in it whatsoever, yet it does contain a lot of truths.

The Bible also quotes Jesus as saying; "You can renew your life by your belief."

I see this as, change the way you think and your life will change, a saying that is now being well used in the 'self-help' industry.

Chapter 12

The Ongoing Journey

I hope that by telling you my story, I have been able to shed some light on that dark space within your mind. I encourage you to keep searching, keep asking questions until you find your own way of releasing yourself from your past negative mindset.

I hope that I have also been able to show you that you *can* make a change. I can only share with you what I have done myself. As a result of fundamentally changing my mind, I am now free from my previous suffering.

You might read one of the books that I have mentioned and not get what I 'got' from it at all. You might be listening to one of the CDs from Ram Dass, Eckhart Tolle, David Hawkins, Bruce Lipton, Wayne Dyer, or Byron Katie and be saying to yourself, "I really don't get this!"

Try acceptance. Just give it a go! Listen or read new things with a still and open mind. Be like a net. Let everything go into your net, and let the net catch what it can and let go of what it can't. Then re-listen and re-read with the same net beside you. As you do, you will gather or 'get' more and more. This will help you create the change you may be looking for.

So in summary, observe your body and then look to your mind. Your body will soon tell you when you are bringing 'no' to a present situation. Your tummy will usually go tight as your body gets ready for the 'fight or flight' mode. Stop right there and ask yourself 'what am I thinking about?'. If you can change the situation, change it. If not, accept that it is the way that it is and then act. If you need help with changing the recorded tape player in your subconscious mind, seek it. Clinical hypnotherapy could be one way to help you and there are now many others such as EFT (Emotional Freedom Technique) and NLP (Neuro Linguistic Programming). You need to find your own path. My intention is to share what worked for me, not to 'sell' anyone the 'perfect potion', or reduce this all down into a 'list of things to do'!

Pay attention to the negative thoughts you may have in your mind or the negative words that you share with others and do a positive exchange. You may find the old stories coming out of your sub-conscious mind that will sabotage all your good conscious intentions and scarily, without you even knowing it! Unless of course you work on being present and the observer of your mind and bat those red buggers out of your court!

Also remember the importance of being conscious as you eat, as well as being conscious of what you eat. Fresh is always best and if you can buy organic, do so!

One thing more I need to impart is that this definitely is an ongoing journey with oneself. Mine is still going! As much as I know now, it never stops my 'past understanding' popping up now and then, or the petticoats of my ego showing from time to time. I too have to be very vigilant, aware, and self-observing, so that I am no longer lost in that negative subconscious part of my mind, not even for a minute. I still feel the suffering of others when I share with them, but then enjoy the freedom that they find when practicing acceptance in each moment.

I know that I will face a very large test in the not too distant future, when my mother passes on. We have come such a long way and now really enjoy our relationship as it is and to have to say 'goodbye' to that will give me great sadness. We chat twice a week on Skype, her with her whisky and me with my coffee, for an hour each time. For her to no longer be behind that Skype button will be hard. When that time comes, I hope I have the courage to celebrate her life by rising above my own suffering, keeping acceptance strongly within me and holding the biggest party in her honor.

With this, I wish you happiness, good health and wellbeing! It won't always be 'good', but when something seems 'bad', it will no longer hold the power over you that it did before. Shakespeare's Hamlet said, "For there is nothing either good or bad, but thinking makes it so." Love his insight!

To those of you that dip into the beginning and end of a book, to decide whether or not to read it, well, and this probably sounds funny coming from a vegetarian, but the meat is in the sandwich baby!

To those of you that have shared my journey through reading this book, thank you for being 'here'. The space within me honors the space within you. This is the meaning of Namaste.

With much love and appreciation,

me

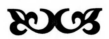